Access the Assessment Programme

To download the Talkabout Assessment of Social Skills software, go to www.routledgelearning.com/tass and click on the 'Gain Access' button.

Answer the question prompt using your copy of the book to download the application.

MORE BRILLIANT PROFESSIONAL RESOURCES FROM BESTSELLING AUTHOR ALEX KELLY!

TALKABOUT

Each practical workbook in this bestselling series provides a clear programme of activities designed to improve self awareness, self esteem and social skills.

Title	Focus	Age-range
Talkabout (3rd edition)	Developing Social Skills for all ages	7+
Talkabout for Children 1 (2nd edition)	Developing Self Awareness and Self Esteem	4–11
Talkabout for Children 2 (3rd edition)	Developing Social Communication	4–11
Talkabout for Children 3 (2nd edition)	Developing Friendship Skills	4–11
Talkabout for Teenagers (2nd edition)	Developing Social and Emotional Communication Skills	11–19
Talkabout for Adults	Developing Self Awareness and Self Esteem in adults	16+
Talkabout Sex and Relationships 1 and 2	Developing Intimate Relationship Skills	11+
Social Skills: Developing Effective Interpersonal Communication	A theory book	n/a

Social Skills: Developing Effective Interpersonal Communication

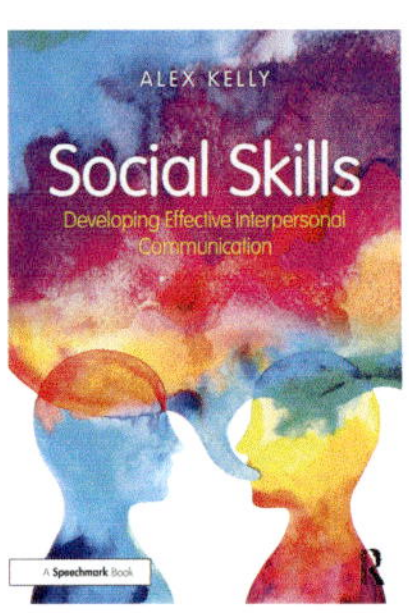

Bestselling author and Speech and Language Therapist Alex Kelly draws on up-to-date theory as well as her years of practical experience to bring you a definitive overview of how social skills develop, what can go wrong, and how people with social difficulties can be supported.

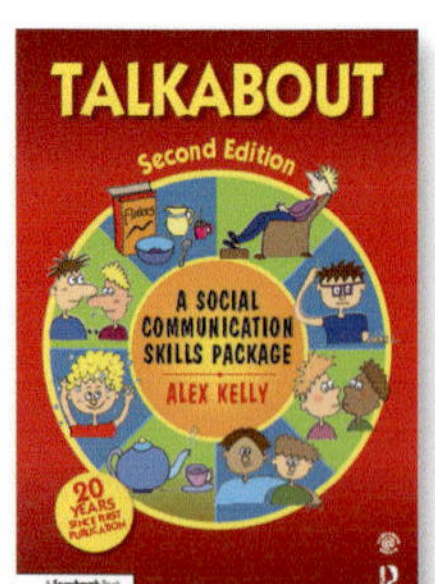

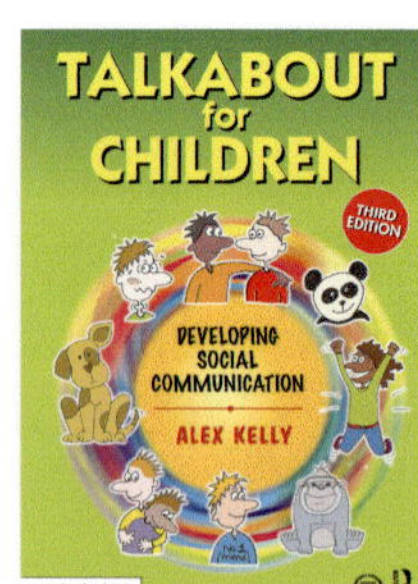

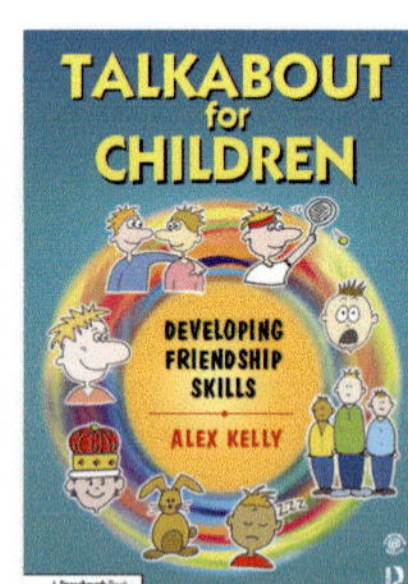

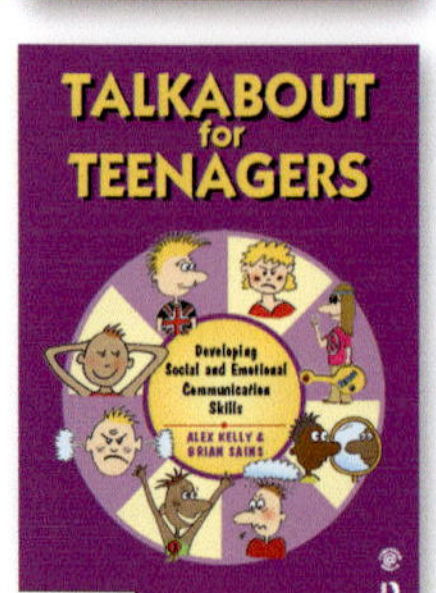

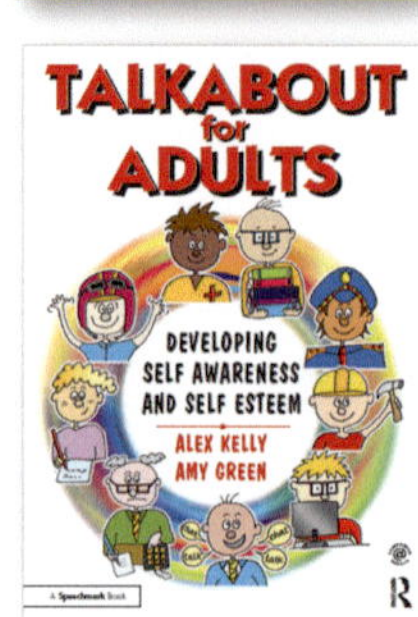

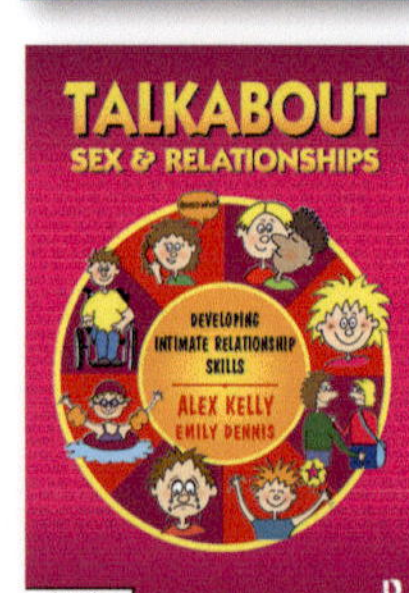

TALKABOUT ASSESSMENT OF SOCIAL SKILLS

The purchase of the TASS manual includes access to the downloadable assessment tool for one user. If you would like to purchase additional downloads for multiple users, or have any queries, please email TASS@tandf.co.uk for more information.

Talkabout Assessment of Social Skills (*TASS*) is an assessment tool using a software programme which allows education and healthcare professionals to input and analyse the assessment of social skills. It gathers information from key sources to provide a holistic view of a person's social communication and uses rating scales to enable quantitative analysis of intervention.

The *TASS* includes a rating of a person's social communication skills (nonverbal, verbal and assertiveness) but also assesses a person within a broader context of social skills including associated factors and quality of life indicators, and an assessment of self-awareness and self-esteem. The *TASS* is divided into five sections:

1. **Initial information**: this section gathers information from significant others and includes reasons for referral, long-term goals, and an initial action plan.
2. **Interview**: a one-to-one interview to assess self-awareness and self-esteem.
3. **Self-rating scale**: an optional part of the assessment, dependent on age and ability, which asks the person to rate their own social communication and identify factors which are important to them.
4. **TASS**: an updated version of the original *Talkabout Assessment Tool* which includes sections on body language, the way we talk, conversational and assertiveness skills.
5. **Summary**: this final part provides summary charts of all sections and areas of high priority.

The *TASS* software programme is supported by an accompanying manual, which includes an overview of the resource and guidelines for each section, in addition to worked examples and photocopiable versions of the digital forms. This complete assessment tool is a valuable resource for anyone working in the area of social communication and is suitable for use by both individual practitioners and teams.

Alex Kelly is the author of the *Talkabout* publications. She worked as a speech and language therapist (SLT) for 37 years, primarily in the area of social communication. She spent 23 years working in the NHS but now runs her own business and spends her time writing and lecturing around the UK and abroad.

Naomi Pearson is a speech and language therapist (SLT) with 24 years' experience working in both the NHS and independent sectors. Naomi is due to complete a PhD in 2024 investigating the effectiveness of the Talkabout programme. She is also the Managing Director of Speaking Space (Romsey) Ltd, based in Hampshire.

TALKABOUT ASSESSMENT OF SOCIAL SKILLS

ALEX KELLY
AND
NAOMI PEARSON

Routledge
Taylor & Francis Group
LONDON AND NEW YORK

Designed cover image: Sarah Hoyle

First published 2024
by Routledge
4 Park Square, Milton Park, Abingdon, Oxon OX14 4RN

and by Routledge
605 Third Avenue, New York, NY 10158

Routledge is an imprint of the Taylor & Francis Group, an informa business

British Library Cataloguing-in-Publication Data
A catalogue record for this book is available from the British Library

ISBN: 978-1-032-77231-8 (hbk)
ISBN: 978-1-032-77230-1 (pbk)
ISBN: 978-1-003-48194-2 (ebk)

DOI: 10.4324/9781003481942

Typeset in Flora Std
by Deanta Global Publishing Services, Chennai, India

Access the Assessment Programme: www.routledgelearning.com/tass

Contents Page

Acknowledgements

The development of the TASS has been a much longer and a far more complicated task than we had ever imagined! And we would not have got it finished without the support of a few individuals.

George Sains – *thank you so much for your hard work and calm attitude to developing the prototype of the TASS. You made the TASS what it is today, and we can't thank you enough for taking time out of your computer science degree deadlines to work with us on this. We think you are so clever and pretty awesome (even though you are Alex's son and so one of us is possibly a bit biased!) and we are forever grateful for your ability to take our initial vision and make it a reality. We have a huge amount of respect for you.*

Nigel Savage – *thank you also to Nigel for taking George's work and developing it further while George finished his degree. You were so good to work with and so patient with us while we tweaked and tweaked!*

Liz Burton and Clare Ashworth – *thank you to our lovely colleagues at Taylor and Francis who have sat through so many meetings on Teams talking about the TASS and helping us to see it through. You have been kind, generous and so encouraging. We couldn't have done it without you.*

Brian Sains and Richard Pearson – *finally we would like to thank our husbands for putting up with us. We know how hard it is to be married to someone who is working hard to get something published and we appreciate your love and support during these last few years.*

Introduction

This section includes

The rationale behind the development of the Talkabout Assessment of Social Skills (TASS)

An introduction to the TASS

Creating a user and client profile

DOI: 10.4324/9781003481942-1

The rationale behind the development of the TASS

Why did the TASS need writing?

Talkabout is a well-established social communication skills programme, popular around the world to help both children and adults develop social communication, self-esteem and friendship skills, and more recently sex and relationship skills. There are currently ten Talkabout books which include intervention programmes for different age groups, and there are also additional resources to supplement intervention, including the Talkabout Boardgame, Talkabout card games, Talkabout Posters and the Talkabout DVD. The Talkabout Assessment CD was published separately in 2009 as another supplementary resource and gave users of Talkabout the ability to assess social skills using a software programme that then generated the 'Talkabout Wheel' – a summary of an individual's social skills profile.

There are several reasons why the authors felt it was time to update the *Talkabout Assessment* (Kelly, 2010). These relate to both the current research in social skills and the practical application and design of the Talkabout wheel.

The following areas have been either updated or included and will be discussed in this section:

1. The hierarchy
2. The rating scale
3. The wider context
4. Social validity

1. The hierarchy

Talkabout was first developed in the early 1990s when the author, Alex Kelly, was working as a speech and language therapist in London, UK. Over a period of four years, she assessed the effectiveness of her social skills interventions and discovered that the success of intervention increased if self-awareness was taught first, and then nonverbal behaviours were taught prior to verbal behaviours, and assertiveness was taught last (Kelly, 1996). This original hierarchy then formed the basis of the first Talkabout book.

In the following years, she became interested in the impact that self-esteem has on social skills and then also the relationship between social skills and friendship skills, and the hierarchy was updated in 2000 to include these two additional areas.

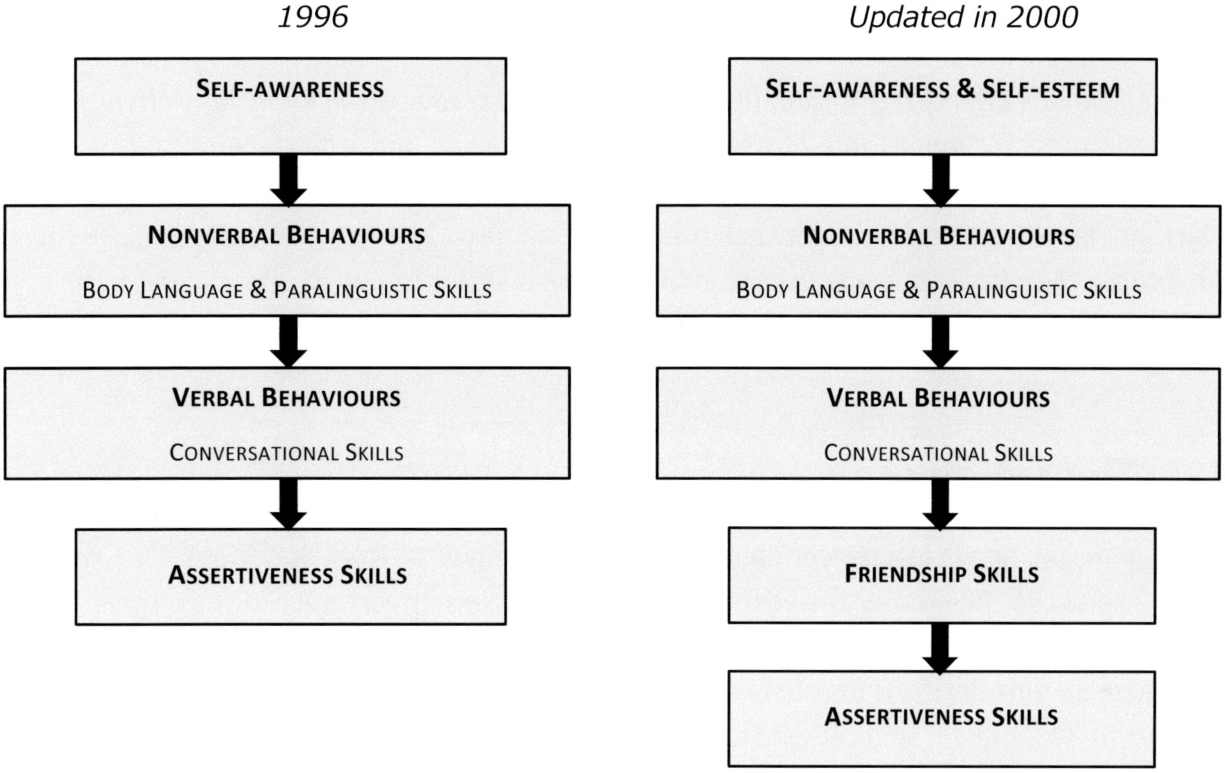

Figure 1.1 *The hierarchy of social skills*

Original (1996) and updated in 2000 to include self-esteem and friendship skills

The Talkabout hierarchy has been developed and extended over the years to reflect increasing knowledge and understanding of the link between self-awareness, self-esteem and social skills, as well as the introduction of friendship skills into the hierarchy. Self-esteem, in particular, is linked to social skills. Firstly, social skills difficulties or differences can be caused by many factors, such as a diagnosis or social background, but can also be caused by 'heightened emotions, other people's behaviour, not knowing the rules, previous experience, a lack of information, illness … and a lack of self-confidence or *low self-esteem*' (Kelly, 2019). If a person has low self-esteem, then it is likely that their social skills will be impacted at some level; and increasing self-esteem can therefore have a positive impact on social communication. Secondly, self-esteem can have a direct impact on our ability to have successful and meaningful relationships.

The original Talkabout Assessment assessed both nonverbal and verbal behaviours under the headings of body language, paralinguistic skills (or the way we talk), conversational skills and assertiveness skills. The assessment of self-awareness and self-esteem (the client interview) was developed separately and was recommended to be completed alongside the wheel at the point of initial assessment. This meant that the assessor completed two separate assessments which *could make the links between them unclear for those using the assessment without having received training.*

Anyone who has attended a Talkabout social skills training course will know how often the trainers impress the importance of working on self-awareness and self-esteem prior to social skills if needs are highlighted within this area. It seemed timely to develop an assessment which guides the assessor through each area of the updated hierarchy, to ensure information is captured together in one assessment, and that the assessor is guided very clearly to the key areas, and order for intervention.

2. The rating scale

The original Talkabout Assessment used a four-point rating scale from 'never good' to 'very good'. The author found over the years that this gives us less opportunity to show small amounts of progress over a shorter period. As a result, Alex devised additional target forms to help teachers and clinicians to rate individual skills on a six-point rating scale from 'skill not present' to 'skill present and consistent'. This enabled us to track progress within *intervention (ratings 1–4) and also to assess whether students have generalised skills* outside *of the intervention (ratings 5–6). These target forms were then used to measure short-term progress and the Talkabout Assessment Wheel was used to summarise the progress over the longer term. However, this all meant a doubling up of assessment data and so it has been recognised for a while that the ideal solution would be to update the Talkabout assessment and the rating scale used.*

The TASS has therefore been updated to a six-point rating scale, meaning that there is no longer a need to do separate short-term and long-term assessments, as the TASS will be able to be used to measure both. This will help with measuring outcomes for intervention.

3. The wider context

The authors also want the assessment to have a holistic profile which draws on literature, specifically regarding current thinking about a definition of social skills and known correlates. The Talkabout hierarchy has a focus on self-awareness and self-esteem and verbal and nonverbal aspects of social communication, as well as assertiveness skills.

Ongoing research in the USA has led to a definition of social and emotional skills called The CASEL Five (CASEL, 2023) which includes self-awareness, self-management, social awareness, relationship skills and responsible decision-making. It is also recognised that there are correlates to social skills, such as 'competing problem behaviours' and 'academic competence' (Gresham & Elliott, 2008). It was felt important to include these in an updated assessment to ensure a holistic assessment of the person's needs.

Research demonstrates that social and emotional learning is linked to quality of life outcomes. Clarke et al., (2021) summarised their findings by stating:

> A growing body of evidence indicates that enhancing social, emotional and behavioural skills (including emotional identification, articulation and regulation; communication skills; conflict resolution skills; behavioural self-regulation; empathy and perspective taking) is a key determinant to young people's mental health and wellbeing, and supports them in achieving positive outcomes in school, work and life.

In addition, the presence of internalising behaviours (e.g., depression, anxiety) or most notably externalising behaviours (e.g., aggression) are associated with increased school absences and have a detrimental effect on the acquisition and performance of social skills and academic achievements (Gresham, 2015).

These known correlates were not measured in the original Talkabout assessment. Therefore, to ensure a holistic assessment takes place, the TASS includes a rating of associated and quality of life factors (see form 1) with the aim to capture any intervention effects with regards to these factors.

4. Social validity

Social validity refers to the extent to which the individual and the key people surrounding that person view the intervention targets as important and acceptable, which is naturally an important consideration in any intervention. The literature also states the importance of measuring social validity pre- and post-intervention (Matson, Matson & Rivet, 2007).

To aid the assessor in considering whether intervention targets are socially valid, the TASS includes the following:

- priority ratings on all assessment forms
- the importance rating on form 3
- the long-term goal stated by the person on form 1

Consideration of this information will ultimately improve the likelihood that intervention will be valid for the individual, and therefore successful.

A note to the assessor ...

Linked to the above point, it is essential that the assessor considers whether social skills intervention is the right intervention for the person at this time. It is important to listen to the person and also to key people in their lives to help you make this decision. The key pieces of information within the assessment which will support this are the self-rating scale, the priority ratings and the long-term goal. There are several points to consider around motivation and underlying reasons for a behaviour.

Motivation

It is essential that the assessor considers motivation. Does the person want to work on social communication? If not, what are their reasons for this? The authors would not work with someone if they were content with who they are and their quality of life. If this is the case, it may be more appropriate to work with other people in the person's life to understand their challenges and support their differences, rather than work with the person themselves.

Underlying reasons for behaviours

It is important to consider other possible reasons for any behaviours that have been highlighted as a need. For example, if a person has been rated a 1 or 2 for fidgeting, it may be appropriate to consider sensory needs, and related strategies to support these. The wording used for the TASS rating scale asks the assessor to consider appropriateness to the situation, with regards to what would be expected of a typical person their age. If a particular behaviour is rated as a potential area of need this doesn't automatically mean that it should be an area to target in your intervention. These ratings must be considered in the context of the whole person and the assessor is advised to ask themselves the following questions:

- *What do the other parts of the assessment show? Does the wider context show you that social communication is impacting their life?*
- *Does the self-rating scale show you that the individual highlights any particular areas as difficult?*
- *Do the priority ratings show you that the individual and key people want support in these areas?*
- *Could there be other explanations for the behaviour such as sensory needs or environmental?*
- *Is their social skills profile associated with a particular diagnosis?*

If your assessment highlights any question marks in any of these areas, you may need to consider these further before you move on to intervention.

In summary

In summary, the aim of the authors in the update of this assessment is to provide a more holistic social skills assessment which draws on the experience and use of the original Talkabout Assessment and the additional resources developed to support the measuring of outcomes, but also on the current literature in social and emotional skills. The authors wanted to develop a tool that is a user-friendly and practical assessment, and which captures information regarding a broad definition of social skills.

An introduction to the Talkabout Assessment of Social Skills (TASS)

An overview of the TASS

The Talkabout Assessment of Social Skills (TASS) is an assessment tool using a software programme which allows you to input and analyse your assessment of social skills. It gathers information from key sources to provide a holistic view of a person's social communication. It also uses rating scales to enable quantitative analysis of intervention.

The TASS includes a rating of a person's social communication skills (nonverbal, verbal and assertiveness) but also assesses a person within a broader context of social skills including associated factors and quality of life indicators, and an assessment of self-awareness and self-esteem.

The TASS includes four assessment forms and a summary section.

TASS: A description of the assessment forms and summary charts

The TASS is divided into four sections and the assessor decides which sections of the assessment are relevant to each person, depending on age and ability.

1. Initial information (f.1). This gathers information from significant others and includes personal information, reason for referral, long-term goal and an initial action plan. There is also a rating of associated factors and quality of life on a rating scale from 1 to 6 ('never' to 'always'), and an ability to rate each factor in terms of priority. This form generates summary charts for both associated factors and quality of life, which can be viewed in the summary section.

2. Interview (f.2). This is a one-to-one interview with the person to assess self-awareness and self-esteem, which is an updated version of the interview from the Talkabout series. The results of this interview are scored using a six-point rating scale and this can be viewed as a bar chart in the summary section.

3. Self-rating scale (f.3). This is an optional part to the assessment, dependent on the person's age and ability. It assesses awareness of their own social communication using a six-point rating scale from 'very difficult' to 'very easy'. It also asks the person to identify any factors which are important to them. This form generates a bar chart which can be viewed in the summary section.

4. TASS (f.4). This is an updated version of the original Talkabout Assessment Tool and includes sections on body language, the way we talk, conversational and assertiveness skills. The TASS uses a six-point rating scale from 'never' to 'always' and a priority rating. This form generates the TASS wheel which can be viewed in the summary section.

5. Summary. In this section the assessor can view the assessment information from all sections, including a summary of areas of high priority. So, in total, there are summary charts for:

    - f.1 Associated factors and quality of life (s.1)
    - f.2 Self-awareness and self-esteem (s.2)
    - f.3 Self-rating scale (s.3)
    - f.4 TASS wheel (s.4)
    - f.1–f.4 Areas of high priority (s.5)

Table 1.1 A summary of the TASS

Assessment			
Assessment	Method	Purpose	Form
1. Initial information	Gathers information from significant others followed by completion of rating scales	• gather personal information • reason for referral • associated factors • quality of life • long term goal	f.1
2. Interview	1:1 interview with person, followed by completion of rating scale	• assess self-awareness • assess self-esteem	f.2
3. Self-rating scale	Individual self-rating	• assess person's awareness of their own social communication	f.3
4. TASS	Assessment of social skills	• assess social skills and to establish a score for body language, the way we talk, conversational and assertiveness skills	f.4
5. Summary charts	n/a	Summary charts of: • associated factors and quality of life • self-awareness and self-esteem • self-rating • social skills • areas of high priority	

Information pages

On every screen/page of the TASS there is an 'i' icon (i) in the corner of the screen which will give the assessor some basic information about that section of the TASS.

Screen resolution

Screen resolution

Please note ... this application works best at a standard display resolution of 1920 × 1080 at 100% so it may be necessary to adjust your settings for optimal use.

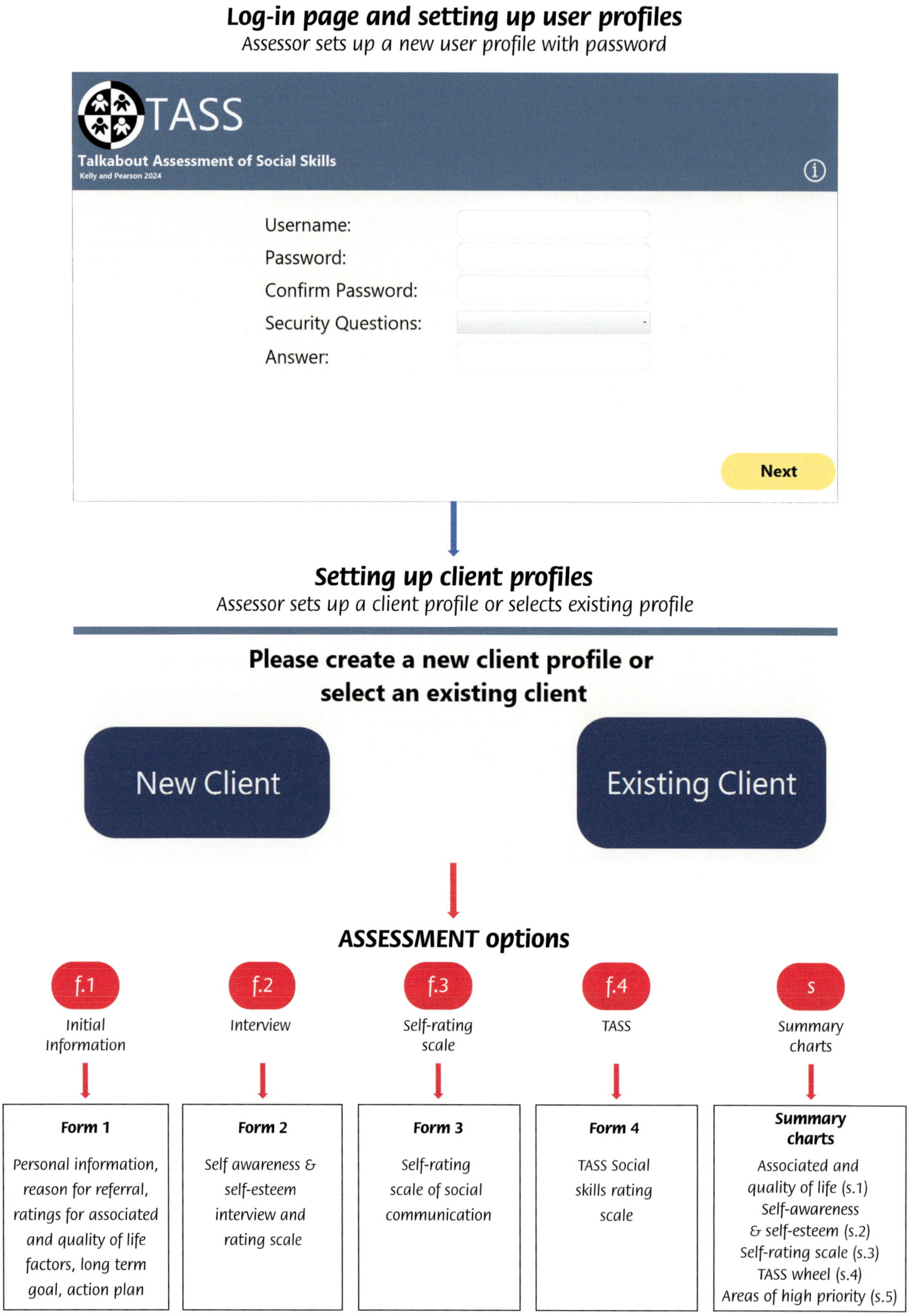

Figure 1.2 The process of the TASS

Creating a user and client profile

Creating a user profile

When you first use the TASS, you will need to create a username and password. This will take you into the main TASS assessment options. You will need to input your username and password each time you open the TASS application.

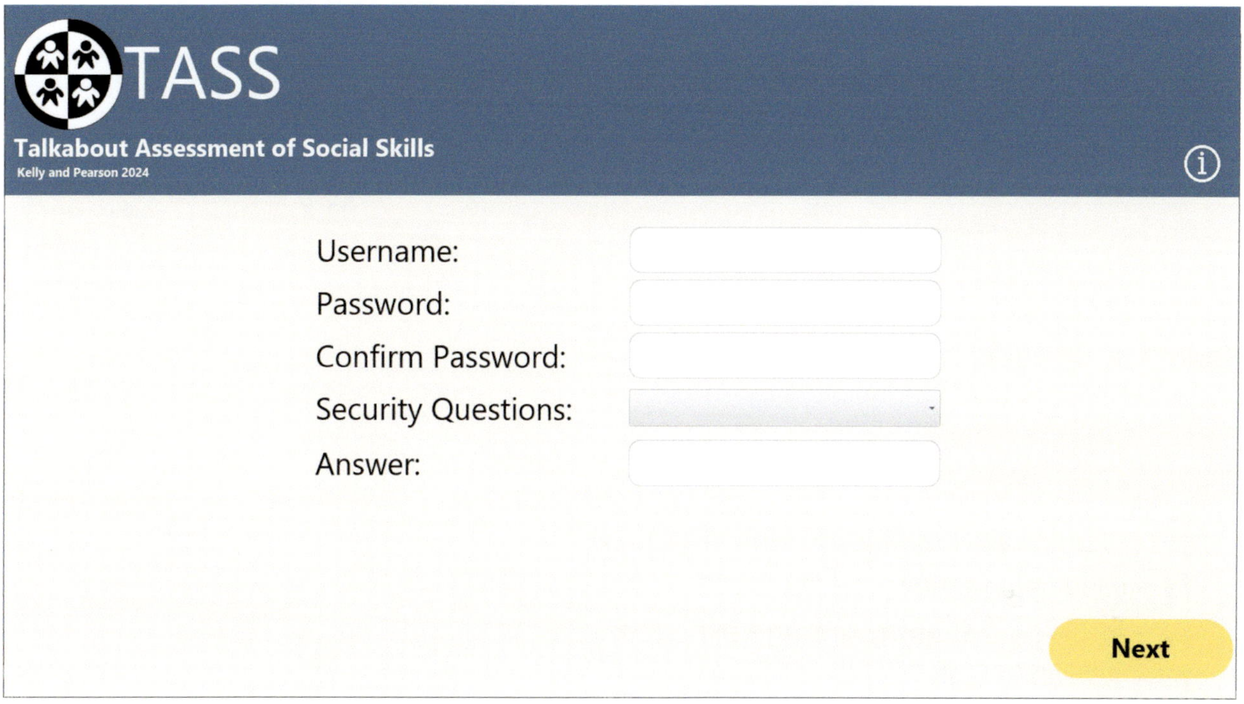

Figure 1.3 *Image of welcome screen*

Creating a client profile

The TASS allows you to set up as many client profiles as are required. You will need to allocate individuals to a group, e.g., 'Year 7' or 'x school', which will mean that you will be able to search for them under that group name. If individuals are not naturally part of a group, you can choose a generic name such as 'nongroup' or 'consultancy'. You will need to select their date of birth from the calendar (rather than type in their date of birth).

Their name and date of birth will now appear in the header of each screen of the TASS.

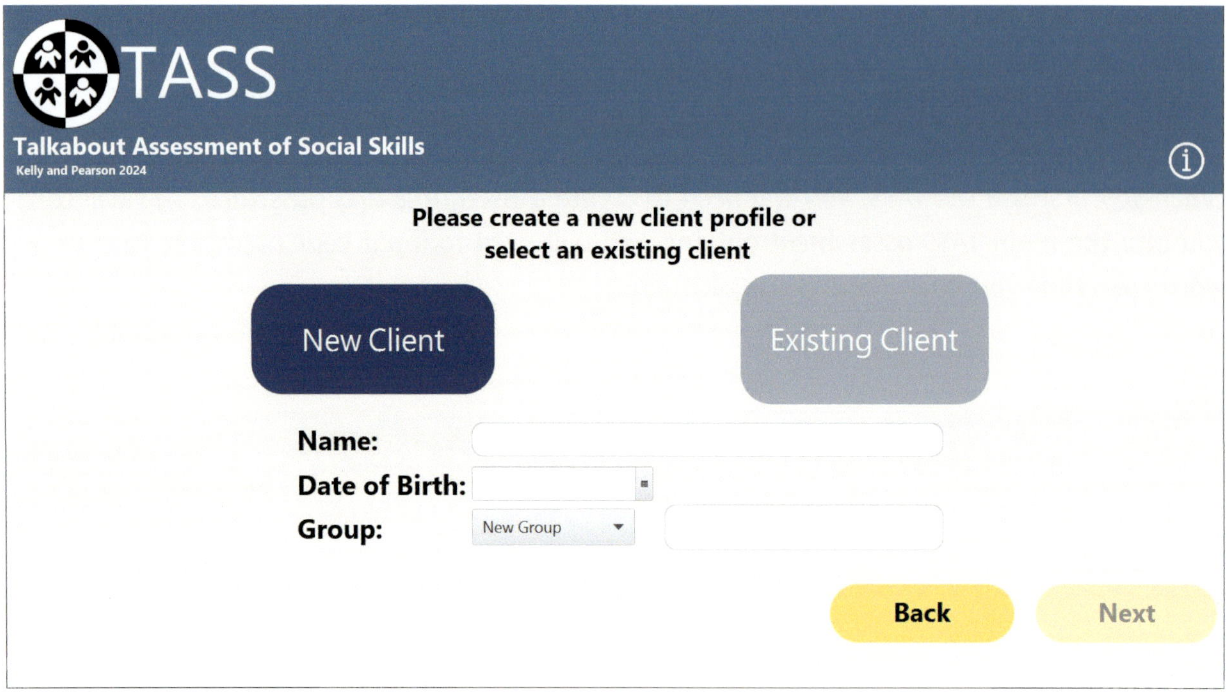

Figure 1.4 *Image of creating a client profile screen*

Assessment options

The TASS is divided into four assessment sections:

- **f.1** – *initial information*
- **f.2** – *interview (self-awareness and self-esteem)*
- **f.3** – *self-rating scale*
- **f.4** – *TASS (social skills)*
- **S** – *summary charts*

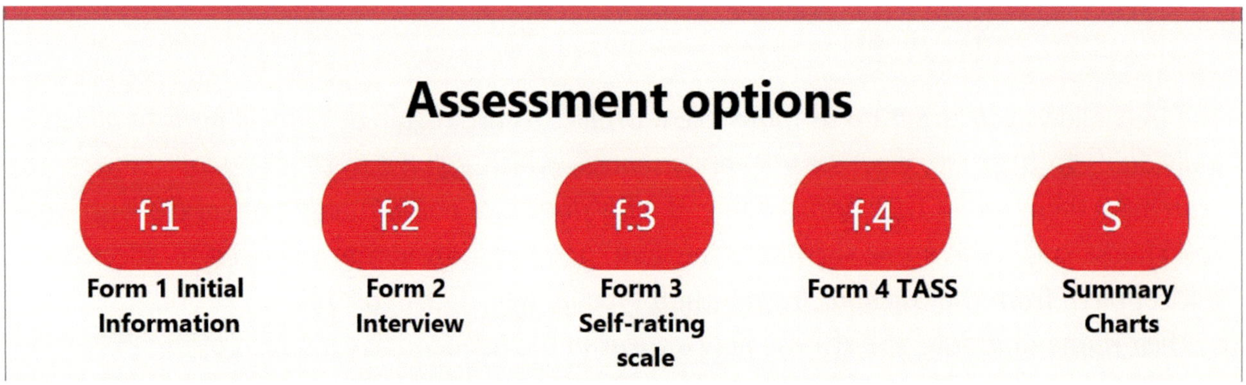

Figure 1.5 *Image of assessment options screen*

Using the software programme and data protection

It is highly recommended that assessors do not store data on the assessment tool for any longer than necessary and that as soon as intervention is completed, that the profile information is exported (print to pdf) and saved in a secure setting.

The user should be aware of their own, and their organisation's responsibilities, for the appropriate use and storage of data and personal information under the General Data Protection Regulations. Please refer to your own or your organisation's GDPR policy to ensure that any data being processed whilst using this package is in accordance with these regulations.

Assessment

This section includes

Assessment main options

Completing f.1 Initial information

Completing f.2 The interview

Completing f.3 The self-rating scale

Completing f.4 The TASS

Summary charts

DOI: 10.4324/9781003481942-2

Assessment options

The assessment (Ax) stage of the TASS has four sections:

f.1 (form 1) Initial information. This form gathers information including personal information, reason for referral, long-term goal and an initial action plan. There is also a rating of associated factors and quality of life, and an ability to rate each factor in terms of priority. This form generates summary charts for both associated factors and quality of life, which can be viewed in the summary section.

f.2 (form 2) Interview. This is a one-to-one interview with the person to assess self-awareness and self-esteem. The results of this interview are scored using a six-point rating scale and this can be viewed as a bar chart in the summary section.

f.3 (form 3) Self-rating scale. This is an optional part to the assessment, dependent on the person's age and ability. It assesses awareness of their own communication using a six-point rating scale. It also asks the person to identify any factors which are important to them. This form generates a bar chart which can be viewed in the summary section.

Assessment main options

Downloading forms. You can download pdfs of the forms onto your computer here. You will be asked to select the folder you wish them to be sent to. They will then appear in a zipped folder named 'TASS assessment forms'.

Completing f.1 INITIAL INFORMATION

f.1 Initial information

This form gathers information from significant others and is designed to be completed by the assessor, the person themselves, or by a significant other, e.g., parent/teacher.

A. Personal information

Completion of this section is self-explanatory. If the client is school aged, then it is useful to have a contact at school who will be involved in the intervention, especially if it is taking place there.

B. Description of person's social skills

Reason for referral: It is useful to have a clear reason for referral in this section. For example, 'support with making new friends' is more useful than 'social skills'. This will provide an insight into the motivation for seeking support with their social communication. If you are aware of the motivation, you can ensure that the intervention is relevant to the person which will result in greater success.

Relevant diagnoses: Social communication differences can be associated with some diagnoses, and so it can be useful to be aware of these prior to intervention.

Examples of situations the person finds difficult: Asking them to think of social situations that the person finds difficult may also help with formulating a clear reason for referral. Again, giving quite specific examples rather than generic ones is more helpful. For example, 'often feels he is left out of the group in the playground' is more useful than 'social situations'. This will provide some practical information regarding the real-life impact of the individual's social communication and what intervention could focus on.

C. Associated factors

Associated factors are scored on a six-point rating scale from 1 (never) to 6 (always). This enables you to observe any potential changes in these areas which may be because of intervention, or alternatively, how these areas may be impacting on the success of intervention. This section also includes a priority rating of each of these factors at the time of assessment.

D. Quality of life

This section highlights some of the quality of life indicators which may be linked to social communication, such as relationship status, friendships and occupational success. Any changes can indicate potential long-term effects of intervention. You will ask the person to rate each of the indicators on a six-point rating scale from 1 (never) to 6 (always), and to indicate the priority of each of the factors.

A summary of these ratings can be viewed in the summary charts section of the TASS, under s.1. This will show the ratings for both associated factors and quality of life (see next section) in two bar charts. These can then be saved, viewed or printed out as a pdf.

E. Action plan

Encouraging the person to consider the aim of intervention helps to focus everyone on the same goal. Again, the more specific this can be the better. So, 'I would like to have a boyfriend' is more helpful than 'to be more sociable'. The long-term goal can be used as an indicator to ensure intervention is socially valid for the person and significant others. This can increase motivation for intervention, and ultimately result in improved intervention outcomes. Listening to the person, and to the important people in their life, is key here.

Based on all the initial information provided, you will agree an action plan which will form the next part of the assessment/intervention process. For example, you may decide to complete the rest of the TASS assessment; or you may already have an idea of an intervention strategy that you would like to initiate such as a social skills group or a 1:1 intervention such as a therapeutic story. It is strongly recommended that if any intervention is planned that all relevant areas of the TASS assessment are completed prior to this, to form a baseline assessment and to ensure intervention is being targeted in the appropriate areas.

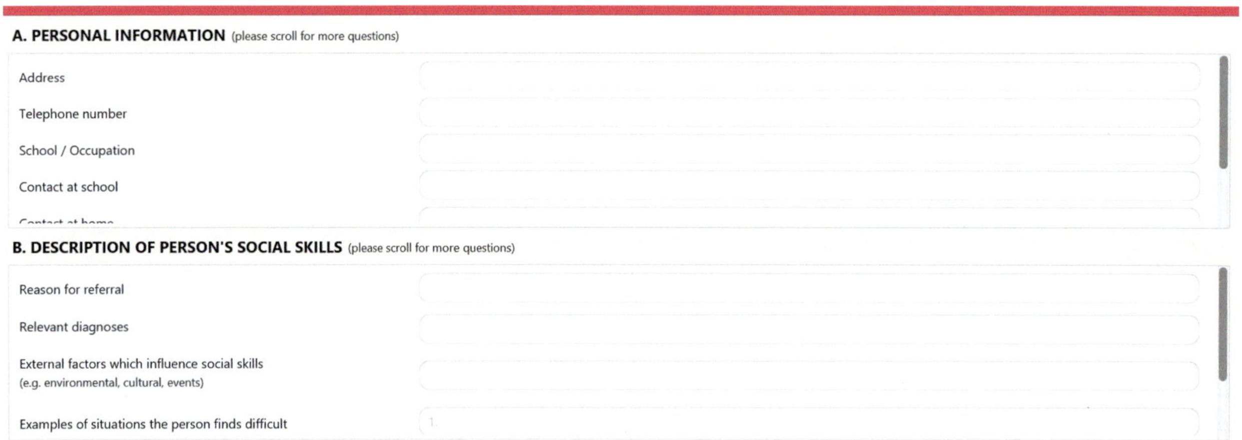

Figure 2.1 f.1 Image of first screen

f.1: Guidelines for scoring

Sections C and D are scored using a six-point rating scale from 'never' to 'always'.

In addition, a priority rating is used for these sections. This is to provide an indication of how important these areas are to the person, and if they could have an impact on the person's social functioning.

On completion of f.1, all quantitative information collated from the rating scales will be presented in bar charts, and factors that have been rated as priority will be summarised in a table. This will form part of your baseline assessment. The assessor may choose some of these as targets for intervention and can then reassess post intervention to evidence progress.

Table 2.1 Rating scale used in f.1

RATING SCALE	What this means …
Never	I never observe this. The person has extensive challenges in this area.
Rarely	I rarely observe this. The person has many challenges in this area.
Occasionally	I occasionally observe this. The person has some challenges in this area.
Sometimes	I sometimes observe this. The person has relative strengths in this area but may still need some support at times.
Mostly	I observe this most of the time. The person has many strengths in this area and does not need support.
Always	I always observe this. The person excels in this area.

f.1: Guidelines for analysing

Table 2.2 *Analysis of f.1 initial information*

f.1: ANALYSING THE INITIAL INFORMATION		
Section	**Take note of …**	**Where does this guide me?**
Personal information	*n/a*	*n/a*
Description of social skills	• *the person's motivation for intervention, i.e., reason for referral, real life situations that the person finds difficult* • *diagnoses or external factors that may impact on intervention*	• *use information on motivation/social validity to decide whether intervention is appropriate and to write relevant intervention targets* • *difficult situations might be used for problem solving* • *consider diagnostic or external factors and how these are impacting the person.* • *is involvement of other professionals required?* • *do other interventions need to be prioritised other than social skills work? e.g., sensory integration* • *does this highlight areas for intervention e.g., emotions work, environmental strategies?*
Associated factors	• *any of these factors which are rated as areas of need and/or a priority for the person*	• *consider if any areas require liaison with other professionals, e.g., teaching staff* • *would 1:1 strategies with regards to behaviour be beneficial (e.g., comic strip, problem solving, social stories)* • *is a behaviour support plan required?*
Quality of life	• *consider any areas which are rated as areas of need and/or a priority for the person*	• *consider how intervention targets can link to improving quality of life for the person (see hierarchy)* • *are any of these areas a long-term goal of intervention?* • *do any other professionals need to be involved?*
Action plan	• *the person's motivation for intervention (long term goal)*	• *use information on motivation/social validity to decide whether intervention is appropriate and to write relevant intervention targets* • *use the long-term goal to explain your rationale for intervention*
Priority rating	• *what are the areas of priority for the person?*	• *are there any priorities highlighted in an area where it would be clinically appropriate to start intervention, considering the hierarchy of social skills? (if so, these should be prioritised first)* • *are any areas of priority likely to impact on the success of intervention, and if so can they be attended to first? (this may require input from other professionals)*

Completing f.2 THE INTERVIEW

f.2 Interview

Overview. This is an informal interview to assess self-awareness and self-esteem. You are asking the person about their likes and dislikes, relationships/friendships, their appearance, feelings, strengths and needs, and qualities. You then rate them on the six-point rating scale at the end. Self-awareness and self-esteem are the first step in the hierarchy of intervention and so it is important to assess this prior to working with someone.

Preparing the person and materials:

- Make the person feel comfortable and as relaxed as possible, so it may be better to make notes or record the session (with the person's consent) and to complete the section on the computer programme later.
- Explain before you start that you are going to ask them a few questions about themselves but if at any time they would prefer not to answer, then that is OK.
- Give the person time to respond before you prompt them. You could help them by repeating back what they have just said to encourage them to say more. For example, 'so you like football…', or you could say 'anything else?' This is then not counted as prompting.
- If they are unable to answer the question, it is possible to prompt them. Initially you may want to prompt them with additional questions/clarifications. This is then noted that they needed a verbal prompt. If you need to use pictures to help them answer, for example giving them a selection of images to choose from, then it is noted that a visual prompt was required. Visual prompts for the following questions are provided in the TASS:
- question 5: what do you look like?
- question 6: how are you feeling?
- question 11: what kind of person are you?

Questions 1 and 2 begin to assess self-awareness and should ease the person into the interview by asking about things they like and enjoy doing and then things they do not like doing. The target for scoring is that they can think of three things for each, so it is a good idea to ask them to think of three things they like/don't like. If it is necessary to prompt them, you could ask 'what about at home – what do you like to do in the evenings?' This would then be marked as a verbal prompt. Visual prompts are not provided for these questions so will need to be prepared by the assessor if necessary.

Question 3 assesses other awareness. The person is asked to talk about someone they know and to say three things about them. You may need to make sure these are accurate so it can be helpful to guide them to talk about someone you both know (e.g., someone at school) so you are able to check accuracy. If they use words like 'nice' or 'lovely', ask them 'what makes them nice?' or 'what do you mean by that?'

Question 4 *asks them to consider what the other person (talked about in the previous question) would say about them. They are asked to think of two things that the other person may say about them. You could say 'imagine they are sitting here, and I ask them to tell me about you, what do you think they would say?'*

Question 5 *continues to assess self-awareness by asking them to say three things about the way they look. These need to be accurate and about their physical appearance. Descriptors such as 'nice hair', 'I have a nose' or 'black trousers and black shoes' would not be counted as they don't give real information about what they look like. In this case, ask for clarification – 'tell me more about your hair'.*

You may want to use visual prompt 1 and there are two versions to choose from. These can be downloaded from the TASS or photocopied from the back of the manual.

Question 6 *begins to assess the person's awareness and understanding of emotions. They are asked to describe how they are feeling and give you some explanation why. If they use words like 'OK' ask them to explain what they mean by that. You may want to use visual prompt 2. There are two versions to choose from. These can be downloaded from the TASS or photocopied from the back of the manual.*

Questions 7 *and* 8 *find out if they can tell you what makes them feel happy/sad and then tell you two things that may help. This is assessing their ability to understand their emotions which is linked to both self-awareness and to the development of self-esteem.*

Question 9 (*and* 4, 11 *and* 12) *assesses the person's awareness of qualities which is part of self-esteem. In question 9, they think of things that they are good at. It is not necessarily relevant if you disagree with what they are saying. For example, if they think they are good at Maths (and you don't think they are), this is still their opinion (and their belief in themselves) and therefore should be assessed as such.*

Questions 10 (*and* 13 *and all the other questions*) *helps to assess the person's self-esteem. Question 10 assesses their ability to consider things that are difficult, which are linked to self-esteem.*

Questions 11 *and* 12 (*and* 4 *and* 9) *assess the person's awareness of qualities which is part of self-esteem. In questions 11 and 12, they consider what kind of person they are. These can be qualities of their personality or more general descriptions about who they are. There is a prompt card to use with question 11 if appropriate. This can be downloaded from the TASS or photocopied from the back of the manual.*

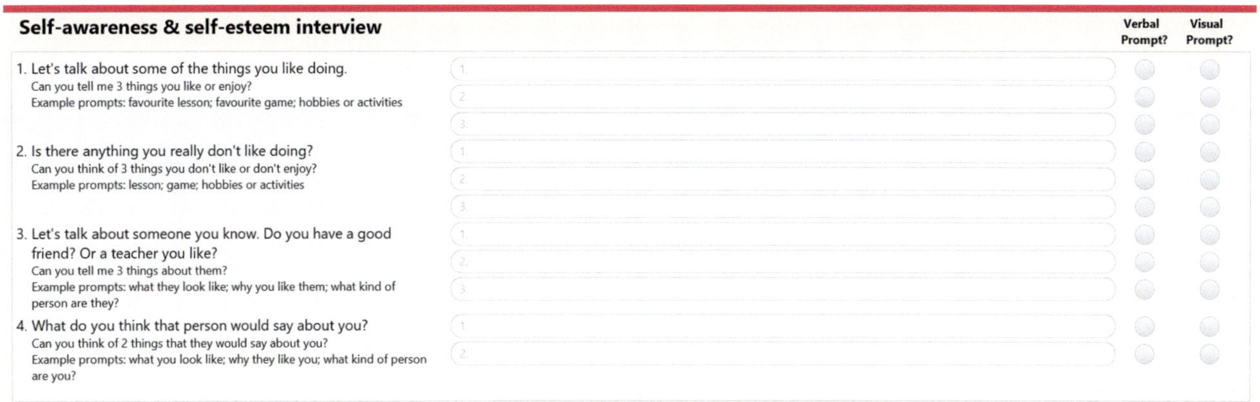

Self-awareness & self-esteem interview — Verbal Prompt? — Visual Prompt?

1. Let's talk about some of the things you like doing.
   Can you tell me 3 things you like or enjoy?
   Example prompts: favourite lesson; favourite game; hobbies or activities
   1. 2. 3.

2. Is there anything you really don't like doing?
   Can you think of 3 things you don't like or don't enjoy?
   Example prompts: lesson; game; hobbies or activities
   1. 2. 3.

3. Let's talk about someone you know. Do you have a good friend? Or a teacher you like?
   Can you tell me 3 things about them?
   Example prompts: what they look like; why you like them; what kind of person are they?
   1. 2. 3.

4. What do you think that person would say about you?
   Can you think of 2 things that they would say about you?
   Example prompts: what you look like; why they like you; what kind of person are you?
   1. 2.

Figure 2.2 *f.2 Image of first screen*

f.2: Further guidelines for completing

Table 2.3 *A description of the questions in f.2*

FORM 2 QUESTIONS	
Question	***A bit more information***
Let's talk about some of the things you like doing	**Questions 1 *and* 2** *begin to assess self-awareness and should ease the person into the interview by asking about things they like and enjoy doing and then things they do not like doing.* *The target for scoring is that they can think of three things for each, so it is a good idea to ask them to think of three things they like/don't like. If it is necessary to prompt them, you could ask 'what about at home – what do you like to do in the evenings?' This would then be marked as a verbal prompt. Visual prompts are not provided for these questions so will need to be prepared by the assessor if necessary.*
Is there anything you really don't like doing?	
Let's talk about someone you know	**Question 3** *assesses other awareness. The person is asked to talk about someone they know and to say three things about them. You may need to make sure these are accurate so it can be helpful to guide them to talk about someone you both know (e.g., someone at school) so you are able to check accuracy. If they use words like 'nice' or 'lovely' ask them 'what makes them nice' or 'what do you mean by that?'*
What do you think that person would say about you?	**Question 4** *asks them to consider what the other person (talked about in the previous question) would say about them. They are asked to think of two things that the other person may say about them. You could say 'imagine they are sitting here, and I ask them to tell me about you, what do you think they would say?'* *This is beginning to assess self-esteem as the person is considering what someone else thinks of him/her.*
Let's talk about the way you look	**Question 5** continues to assess self-awareness by asking them to say three things about the way they look. These need to be accurate and about their physical appearance. Descriptors such as 'nice hair', 'I have a nose' or 'black trousers and black shoes' would not be counted as they don't give real information about what they look like. In this case, ask for clarification – 'tell me more about your hair'. *You may want to use visual prompt 1* and there are two versions to choose from (see pages 26 and 27). These can be downloaded from the TASS or photocopied from the back of the manual.

FORM 2 QUESTIONS	
Question	**A bit more information**
How are you feeling today? *Let's talk about your feelings more …* *What helps you when you are feeling sad or angry or worried?*	**Questions 6, 7 and 8** assess the person's awareness and understanding of emotions. In question 6, they are asked to describe how they are feeling and to explain why. If they use words like 'OK' ask them to explain what they mean by that. *You may want to use visual prompt 2.* There are two versions to choose from (see pages 28 and 29). In questions 7 and 8 find out if they are able to tell you what makes them feel happy/sad and then tell you two things that may help. This is assessing their ability to understand their emotions which is linked to both self-awareness and to the development of self-esteem.
What are you good at?	**Question 9 (and 4, 11 and 12)** assesses the person's awareness of qualities which is part of self-esteem. In question 9, they think of things that they are good at. It is not necessarily relevant if you disagree with what they are saying. For example, if they think they are good at Maths (and you don't think they are), this is still their opinion (and their belief in themselves) and therefore should be assessed as such.
Is there anything you find difficult?	**Questions 10 (and 13, and all the other questions)** helps to assess the person's self-esteem. Question 10 assesses their ability to consider things that are difficult, which is linked to self-esteem.
What kind of person do you think you are? *Tell me the best thing about being you*	**Questions 11 and 12 (and 4 and 9)** assess the person's awareness of qualities which is part of self-esteem. In questions 11 and 12, they consider what kind of person they are. These can be qualities of their personality or more general descriptions about who they are. *There is a prompt card to use with question 11 if appropriate* (see page 30).
If you could change one thing about being you, what would it be?	**Questions 13 (and 10, and all the other questions)** helps to assess the person's self-esteem. Consider the reality of their answer, i.e., have they chosen something realistic or unattainable.
Is there anything you would like to ask me?	**Question 14** is used to bring the interview to a close and to give someone the opportunity to ask any questions about what is happening. The answer to this question does not necessarily inform your scoring or analysis but may, depending on the answer.

VISUAL PROMPT 1: What do you look like? (1)

This is the first prompt card to use with question 5. For example, can the person tell you what they look like with the visual prompt 'hair colour'?

What do you look like? (1)

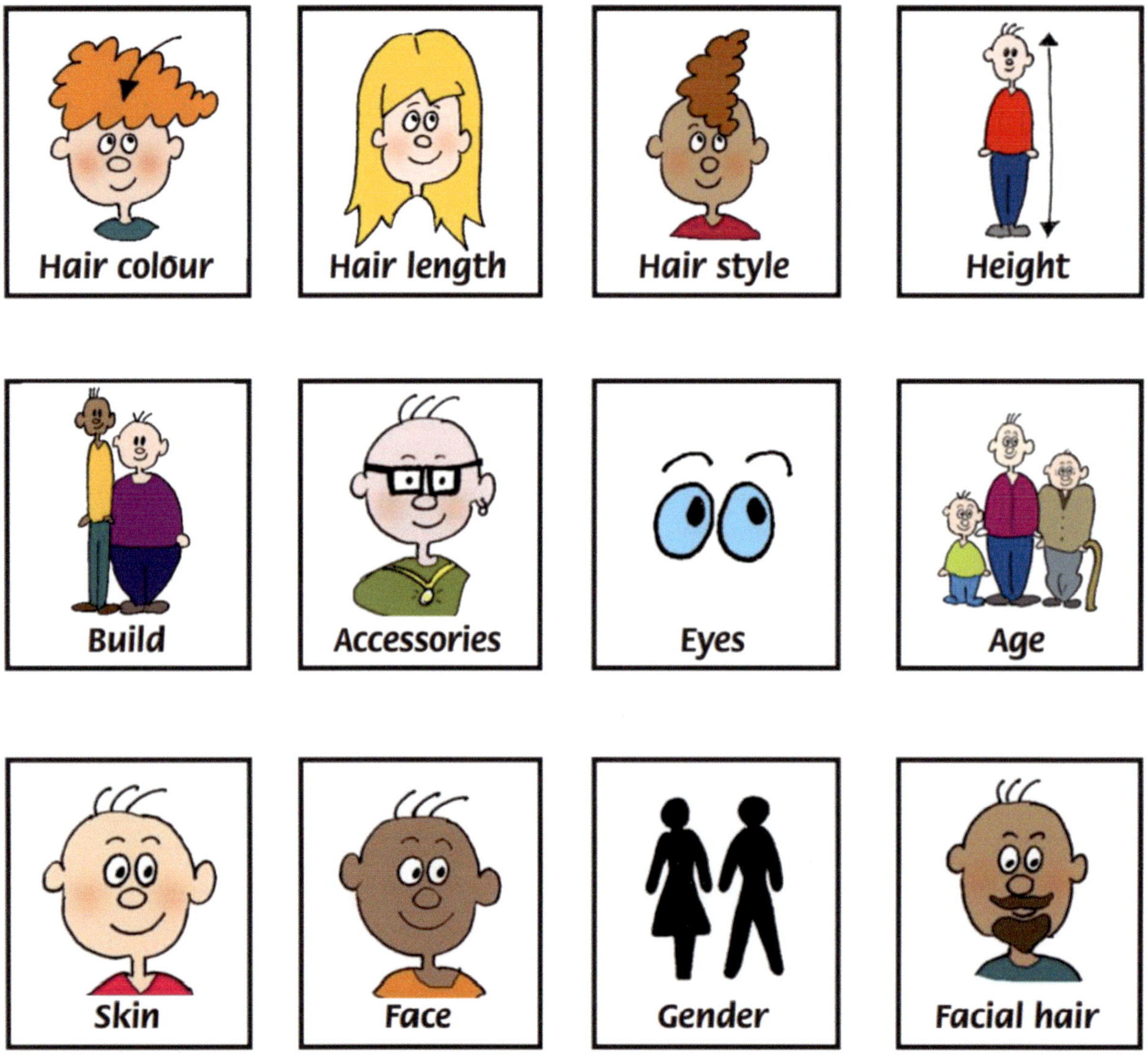

Prompt 1 Question 5

VISUAL PROMPT 1: What do you look like? (2)

This is the easier prompt card to use with question 5. For example, can the person tell you what colour their hair is with the prompts 'brown, blond, black or red'?

What do you look like? (2)

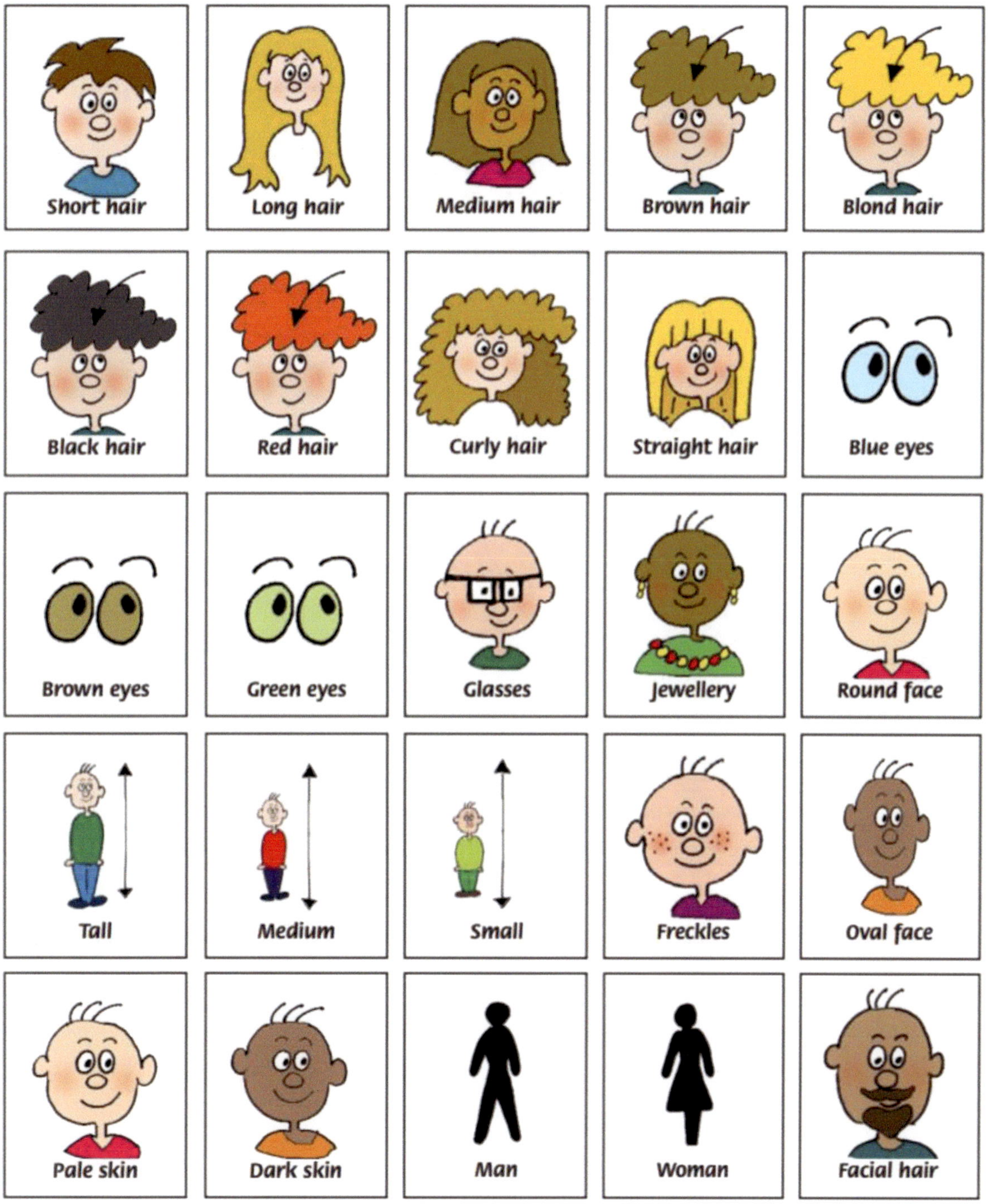

Prompt 1 Question 5

VISUAL PROMPT 2: How are you feeling? (1)

This is the easier prompt card to use with question 6. For example, can the person tell you how they are feeling using the visuals below?

How are you feeling? (1)

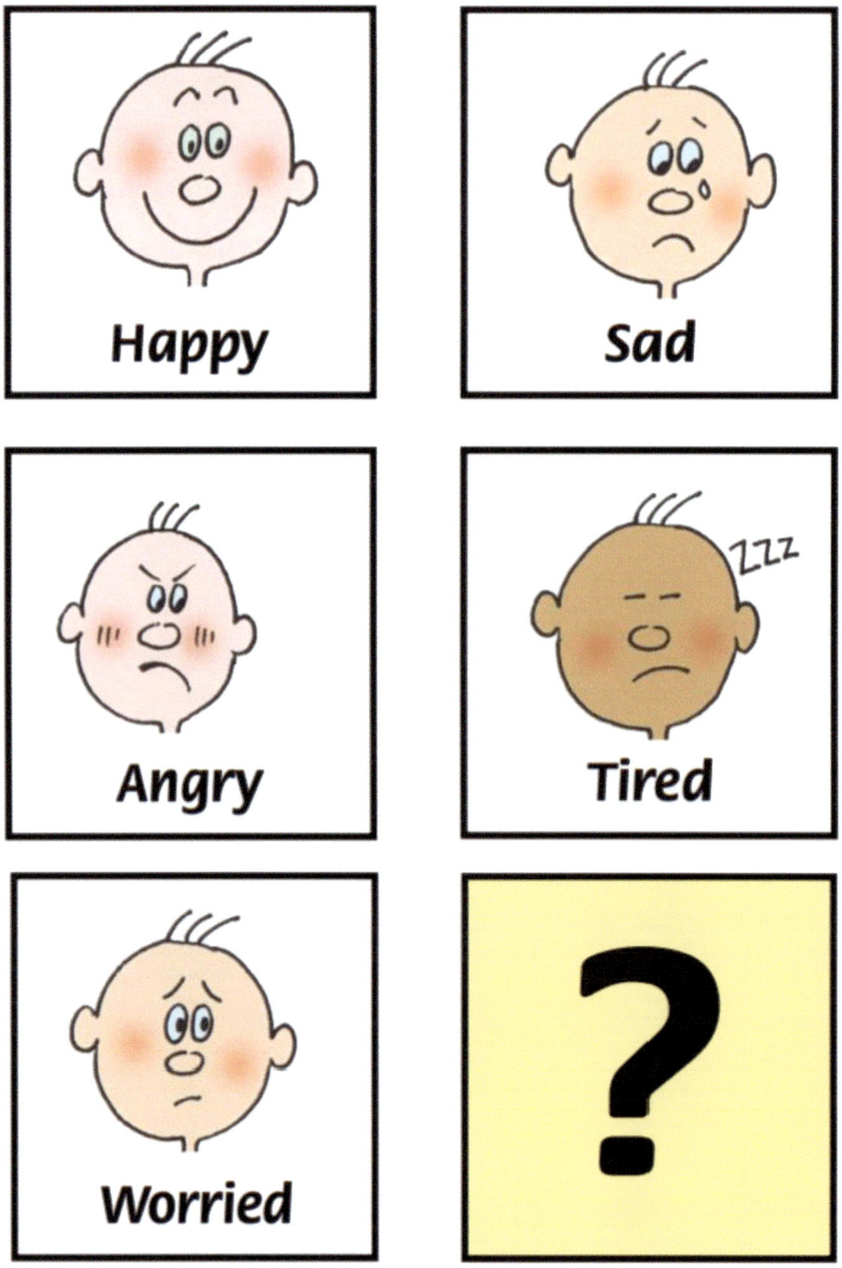

Prompt 2 Question 6

VISUAL PROMPT 2: How are you feeling? (2)

This is the harder prompt card to use with older or more able clients with question 6. Can the person tell you how they are feeling using the visuals below?

How are you feeling? (2)

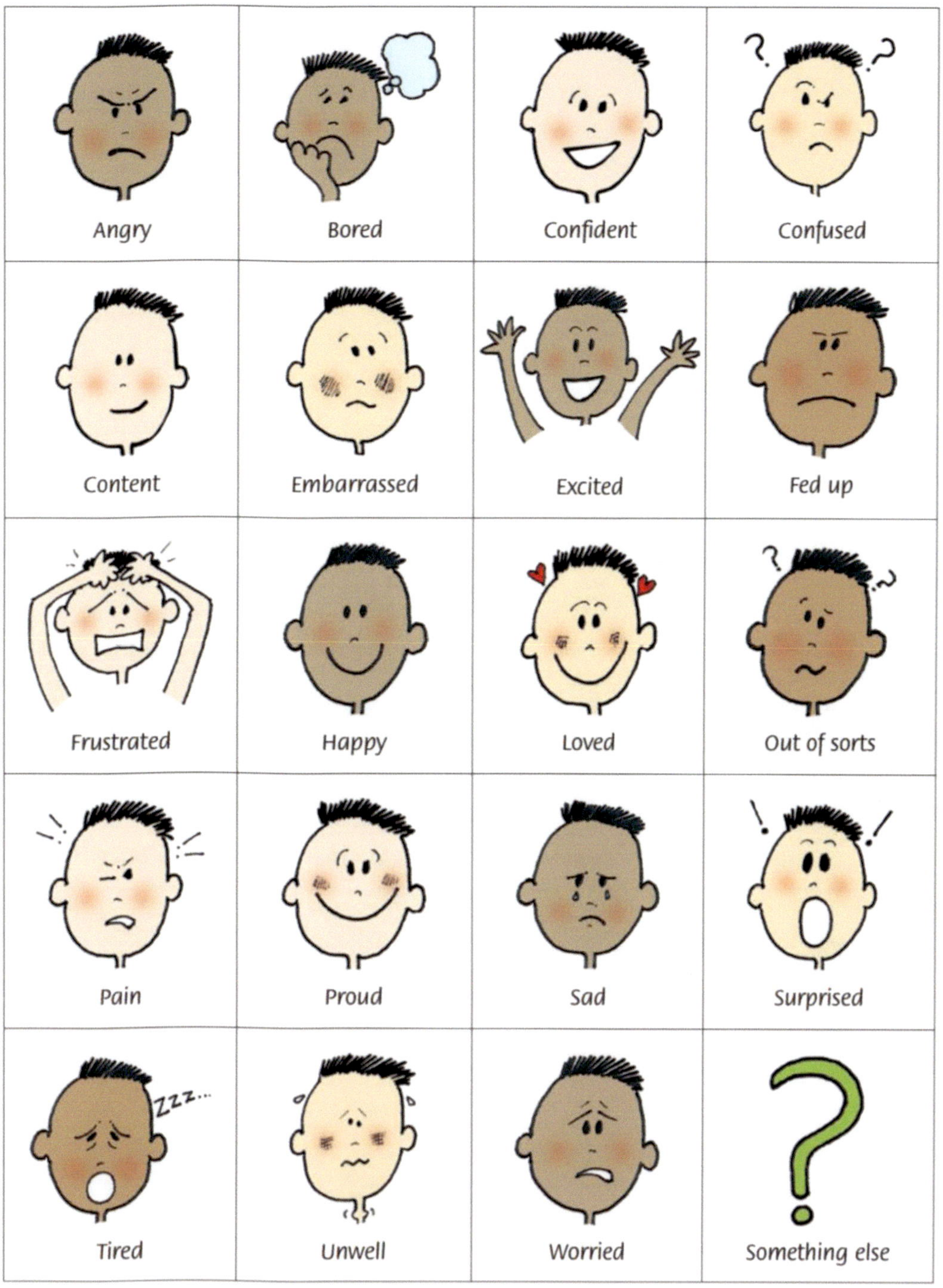

Prompt 2 Question 6

VISUAL PROMPT 3: What are you like?

This is the prompt card to use with question 11. For example, can the person tell you what kind of person they are by choosing three to five pictures below?

What are you like?

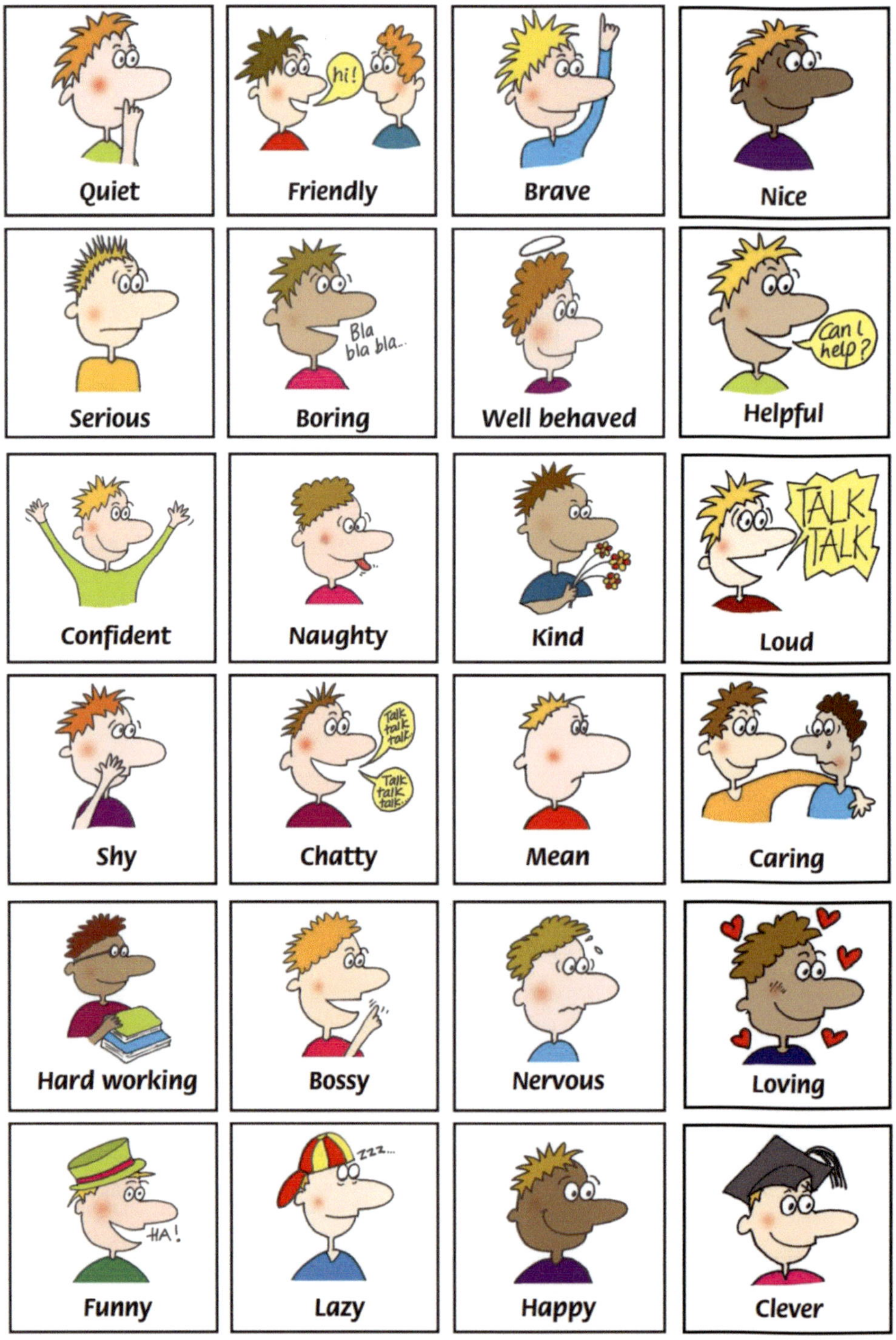

f.2: Guidelines for scoring

f.2 is scored using seven self-awareness and self-esteem targets. Self-awareness is assessed through questions 1, 2, 3 and 5. Awareness and understanding of emotions is assessed through questions 6, 7 and 8. Self-esteem is assessed through all the answers throughout the interview but in particular through questions 4, 9, 11 and 12, and also through questions 10, 13 and 14 where the assessor is looking at whether the person talks positively about themselves.

These targets reflect the areas worked on in the Talkabout resources (see *Talkabout for Children: developing self-awareness and self-esteem*, Kelly, 2018a; *Talkabout for Teenagers*, Kelly & Sains, 2009 and *Talkabout for Adults*, Kelly & Green, 2014).

Table 2.4 The areas, targets and questions in f.2

Area	Target	Question(s)
Self/other awareness	Likes and dislikes	1 and 2
	Other awareness	3
	Personal awareness	5
Emotions	Expressing emotions	6
	Understanding emotions	7 and 8
Self-esteem	Qualities and strengths	4, 9, 11 and 12
	Self-esteem	10 and 13 (and all other questions)

Having completed the interview, the assessor scores the person on these targets using a six-point rating scale.

So, the person will score a '1' if they were unable to meet the target (even with prompting). If they were able to achieve the target but required prompting, then you will score them either a '2' or a '3' depending on how much prompting was needed. If they met the target, you would score them from between a '4' to a '6' depending whether they are able to use this behaviour outside of the situation.

It may not be possible to rate above a score of 4 until the assessor has discussed the findings of the interview with someone who knows the person well or until the assessor can test their skills outside of the structured interview. For example, if they can tell the assessor what they are feeling and why (question 4), then a score of 4 would be given. But if the assessor knows that they are also able to do this in everyday situations, then a score of 5 or 6 would be given.

Table 2.5 *The six-point rating scale used in f.2*

Rating scale	**What this means ...**
1 **No, *never*** *even with lots of support*	*The person is unable to meet the target even with prompting*
2 ***Yes, but rarely*** *and only with lots of support*	*The person needed lots of prompting (either verbal or visual) to achieve the target*
3 **Yes, occasionally** *or with some support*	*The person needed some prompting (either verbal or visual) to achieve the target*
4 **Yes, sometimes** *or in familiar situations only*	*The person was able to do this, but it is likely that this was because it was a structured situation*
5 **Yes, mostly** *but not always*	*The person was able to achieve this, but it is likely that this may not always be the case*
6 **Yes, *always***	*The person is confident in reaching this target and all other relevant people agree that this is not an area of need*

These scores form a baseline score and are shown as a bar chart on the summary page s.2. Once the rating scale has been completed, consider what the top priorities are for that section and what the top areas for intervention would be for the person.

Challenges in this area would indicate that this is where intervention may need to start as it will impact on social communication skills.

Table 2.6 *Scoring f.2*

f.2: SCORING THE INTERVIEW				
Area	**Skill**	**Target**	**Questions**	**Summary**
Self/other awareness	Likes and dislikes	Is able to describe three things they like and three things they dislike	1 and 2	✓ gives three likes ✓ gives three dislikes
	Other awareness	Is able to describe someone else using at least three descriptive words	3	✓ gives three accurate, descriptive words about someone else
	Personal awareness	Is able to describe the way they look using at least three descriptive words	5	✓ gives three accurate, descriptive words about the way they look
Emotions	Expressing emotions	Is able to tell you how they are feeling and why	6	✓ can describe how they are feeling and why.
	Understanding emotions	Is able to tell you two things that shows some insight into what makes them feel happy/sad or something that helps	7 and 8	✓ can think of at least one situation that makes them feel happy for example. ✓ can think of two ideas of what could help if they are feeling angry, sad or worried
Self-esteem	Qualities and strengths	Is able to say three qualities/strengths about themselves	4, 9, 11 and 12	✓ gives three qualities or strengths about themselves in total across these questions
	Self-esteem	Is able to talk positively about themselves and give at least three positive descriptors	All	✓ gives three positive descriptors about themselves across the whole assessment ✓ talks positively about themselves using positive language across the whole assessment

f.2: Guidelines for analysing

The first consideration is whether the person is showing strengths or challenges in their self-awareness and self-esteem. Strengths in this area would indicate that you are able to prioritise work on their social skills. **Challenges in this area would indicate that this is where you will want to start work**.

Depending on the age of the person you could look at the following resources:

- *Talkabout for Children: developing self-awareness and self-esteem*
- *Talkabout for Teenagers* (level 1)
- *Talkabout for Adults*

People with low self-esteem may also have challenges in coping with their emotions (questions 6–8) so emotions should be included in self-awareness and self-esteem work. You may want to look at some of the activities from *Talkabout Theory of Mind*.

Secondly, it is interesting to note the extent of their challenges which will indicate the type of intervention and the speed with which you will be able to work through the programme.

Table 2.7 Rating and type of intervention

RATING SCALE	What this means …	What this means for intervention …
1 **No, never** even with lots of support	The skill has possibly never been learnt	The person may benefit from being taught the skill and the rules where necessary
2 **Yes, but rarely** and only with lots of support	The skill has possibly never been learnt (if prompting was significant) or the person has learnt the skill but has not learnt to use it	The person may benefit from being taught the skill (as above)
3 **Yes, occasionally** or with some support	The person has learnt the skill but has not learnt to use it effectively or to generalise it	The person may benefit from learning and practising the skill within a structured situation
4 **Yes, sometimes** or in familiar situations only	The person has learnt the skill but has not learnt to generalise it	The person may benefit from support to practise the skill in different situations
5 **Yes, mostly** but not always	The person has learnt the skill but has not learnt to generalise it in every situation	The person may benefit from support to practise the skill in a wider range of situations
6 **Yes, always**	This indicates a *strength*	The person may no longer benefit from intervention in this area

Completing f.3 THE SELF-RATING SCALE

f.3 Self-rating scale

f.3 is an optional part of the assessment which the person completes themselves. This self-rating scale includes ratings related to a few of the associated factors, self-awareness and self-esteem, and some of the social skills behaviours assessed on the TASS rating scale (f.4). There is a six-point rating scale from 'very difficult' (1) to 'very easy' (6), and the person is also asked which behaviours are very important to them.

Guidelines for completing

This form should only be completed if you feel it is appropriate for the person. You may want to consider the age, cognitive skills and level of comprehension and expression of the person. If they are unable to understand the rating scale, then it will not be a meaningful assessment.

The following steps will help with the reliability:

1. *Complete the form in a quiet 1:1 situation free from distractions*
2. *Ensure the person understands the rating scale – you may want to practise with an unrelated item, e.g., 'Maths' – 'how easy or difficult do you find that? How would you rate that?'*
3. *If it helps, you can draw the rating scale out on a big piece of paper so the person can point to their answers.*
4. *Once they understand the rating scale, try the first couple at the beginning of the rating scale together.*
5. *Ask the person to tell you if they need some help to understand any of the statements. Thinking of examples which illustrate the point can help.*
6. *You can also check their understanding periodically throughout the assessment by asking questions such as – 'what do you think we mean by that?'*
7. *If they consistently do not understand what you are asking, you may choose to stop the assessment.*
8. *A person may appear to understand what is being asked but rate themselves highly throughout. Conversely, a person might give themself very low ratings. If you do not agree with their self-rating, you should not question it. The purpose of this assessment is to understand the person's perspective so they should not be corrected, or their ratings re-negotiated.*
9. *This assessment can be completed in five minutes, or it may take longer if discussion takes place. You can always choose to take a break halfway through.*

Guidelines for analysing

The self-rating scale can add a wealth of information to the holistic assessment of a person's social communication skills profile, and unless there is a clear rationale as to why this should not be completed, it will undoubtedly contribute to a rich and thorough assessment of the person's needs and will also help to inform your intervention plan.

Questions 1–3: Associated factors and quality of life

- *these are known associated and quality of life factors and can be compared to the ratings in f.1 questions C2 and D4*

Questions 4–9: Self-awareness and self-esteem

- *does the person demonstrate low self-awareness and self-esteem (f.2)?*
- *do their answers raise any questions when compared to the ratings in f.2?*

Questions 10 and 11: Body language

- *compare ratings of the same area on the TASS (f.4, questions 1–8)*

Question 12: The way we talk

- *compare ratings of the same area on the TASS (f.4, questions 9–13)*

Questions 13–17: Conversational skills

- *compare ratings of the same area on the TASS (f.4, questions 14–21)*

Question 18: Assertiveness skills

- *compare ratings of the same area on the TASS (f.4, questions 22–9)*

Priority rating

- *ask the person to choose a few that are really important to them*
- *this may give some indication of the person's motivation and social validity, which will be helpful when considering intervention*
- *are there any priorities highlighted in an area where it would be clinically appropriate to start intervention, considering the hierarchy of social skills?*
- *if the person has highlighted priority areas in a clinical area where it is not appropriate to start work, can they be supported to understand how planned intervention targets will help the person to reach their long-term goal?*

When f.3 is completed, the ratings will be displayed in a bar chart format. Any social skills which the person has rated as important will be displayed in a list in the summary charts.

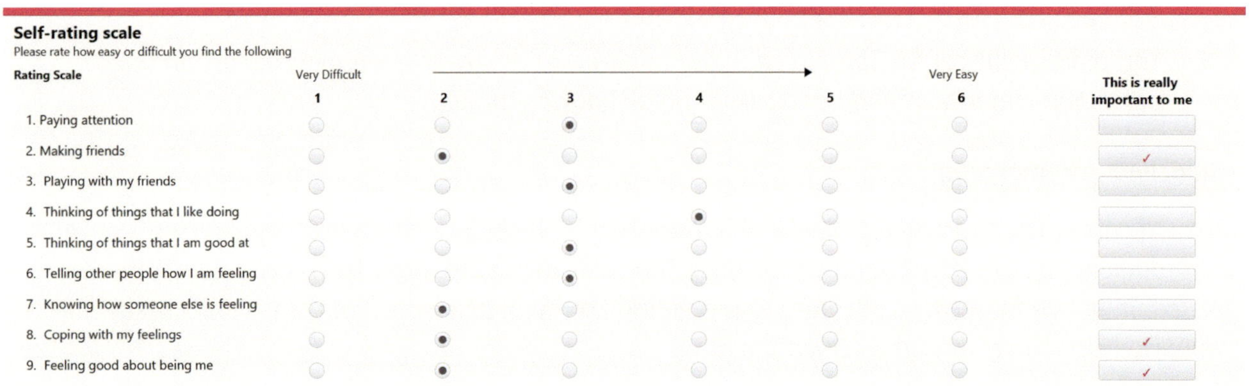

Self-rating scale

Please rate how easy or difficult you find the following

Rating Scale	1 (Very Difficult)	2	3	4	5	6 (Very Easy)	This is really important to me
1. Paying attention			●				
2. Making friends		●					✓
3. Playing with my friends			●				
4. Thinking of things that I like doing				●			
5. Thinking of things that I am good at			●				
6. Telling other people how I am feeling			●				
7. Knowing how someone else is feeling		●					
8. Coping with my feelings		●					✓
9. Feeling good about being me		●					✓

Figure 2.3 *f.3 Image of first screen*

f.3: Guidelines for scoring

There are two elements to the scoring of this assessment:

1. *The rating scale: The person is asked to rate themselves on 18 behaviours on a six-point rating scale from 'very difficult' (1) to 'very easy' (6).*
2. *Priority ratings: Once the rating scale has been completed by the person (if appropriate) ask them to consider which areas are most important to them, and to highlight these in the box labelled 'this is really important to me'. They may need to look back over the rating scale to remind them of the questions. If the person chooses lots of areas as a priority, it might be useful to ask what they would choose to work on right now if they could pick three top priorities. Again, there is no limit to the number which can be chosen.*

f.3: Guidelines for analysing

The self-rating scale can add a wealth of information to the holistic assessment of a person's social skills profile, and unless there is a clear rationale as to why this should not be completed, it will undoubtedly contribute to a rich and thorough assessment of the person's needs and will also help to inform the assessor's intervention plan.

Some points to consider when analysing the results would be:

- *Are there some potential areas of need for the person i.e. which areas did they rate as most difficult?*
- *Does the person either rate themselves to be consistently low or consistently high and what might the reasons for this be?*
- *Where any needs are highlighted, are these in the same area of the hierarchy? For example, does a person find all areas of self-esteem very difficult?*
- *How do the person's ratings compare to other parts of the assessment, i.e. the assessor's ratings in the interview and TASS? Where are the areas of agreement or discrepancy and what might be the reasons for this?*
- *Based on the person's own judgements compared to others in forms 2 and 4, what would be the assessor's view of the person's self-awareness? Does the assessor need to carry out some observations to determine this?*
- *Which areas does the person view as the most important? Are these the same as the areas of need, or are they different?*

- *How do the importance ratings compare to the priority ratings in forms 1, 2 and 4? Does everyone agree about the areas of priority and therefore should intervention start here? If there are areas of disagreement, why is this? Is the person demonstrating low self-awareness and therefore should intervention start here? Is more information needed about how they present in different environments?*
- *What are the top priorities for this person, and based on the rest of the assessment is this an appropriate place to start intervention?*

Table 2.8 gives specific guidance for each section of the assessment.

Table 2.8 *Analysis of f.3 self-rating scale*

f.3: ANALYSING THE SELF-RATING SCALE		
Questions	***Take note of …***	***Where does this guide me?***
Questions 1–3: associated factors and quality of life	These are known associated and quality of life factors	Compare their answers to the ratings in f.1 questions C2 and D4
Questions 4–9: self-awareness and self-esteem	Does the person demonstrate low self-awareness and self-esteem (interview f.2)?	Do their answers raise any questions in relation to self-awareness or self-esteem when compared to f.2 ratings? Use f.2 to decide if this is an appropriate place to start intervention. Consider the hierarchy when setting intervention targets – if the person demonstrates needs in this area the priority should be to start here
Questions 10–11: body language	How does this compare to ratings of the same area on the TASS (f.4, questions 1–8)?	Consider the hierarchy when setting intervention targets – remember that body language is prioritised for intervention after self-awareness and self-esteem has been developed (if appropriate)
Question 12: the way we talk	How does this compare to ratings of the same area on the TASS (f.4, questions 9–13)?	Consider the hierarchy when setting intervention targets – remember that the way we talk is a nonverbal skill and is prioritised for intervention after body language
Question 13–17: conversational skills	How does this compare to ratings of the same area on the TASS (f.4, questions 14–21)?	Consider the hierarchy when setting intervention targets – remember that verbal skills are developed after nonverbal skills
Question 18: assertiveness	How does this compare to ratings of the same area on the TASS (f.4, questions 22–9)?	Consider the hierarchy when setting intervention targets. Remember that assertiveness is the last thing to teach in the hierarchy, and so the person should have enough underpinning skills in order to learn this
All questions/ priority ratings	Are there any priorities highlighted where it would be clinically appropriate to start intervention, considering the hierarchy of social skills? If the person has highlighted priority areas in a clinical area where it is not appropriate to start work, can they be supported to understand how planned intervention targets will help the person to reach their long-term goal?	Priority areas for intervention would be those that are marked as a priority and are also an appropriate place to begin intervention in relation to the hierarchy of social skills. Consider providing support to understand why intervention is not starting at a priority area if this is the case, to ensure motivation for intervention remains, and how intervention is linked to the person's long-term goal

Completing f.4 The TASS

f.4 TASS

The TASS is the main assessment of social skills and includes sections on body language, the way we talk, conversational and assertiveness skills. This form should be completed by you, not the person or parent. Use your observations and information from other people to score the person on each skill using the descriptions in the manual and the six-point rating scale in terms of appropriateness to a situation: from 'never' to 'always'. Remember to rate according to what is appropriate for them in terms of age and culture. This then generates the TASS wheel, which is viewed in the summary section.

The six-point rating scale

RATING SCALE	*What this means when scoring the TASS*
1 **Never**	*The person is unable to do this even with lots of support/prompting.*
2 **Rarely**	*The person is only able to do this on rare occasions and/or needs lots of prompting (either verbal or visual).*
3 **Occasionally**	*The person is only able to do this occasionally and/or needs some support (either verbal or visual).*
4 **Sometimes**	*The person is sometimes able to do this but only in familiar situations, so they have not learnt to generalise the skill outside of structured or highly familiar settings.*
5 **Mostly**	*The person is mostly able to do this, but they may be unable to in some situations.*
6 **Always**	*The person is confidently able to do this in all situations.*

The four sections of the TASS include:

Body language

There are eight behaviours in total to assess someone's body language using the descriptions in the manual (below) and the six-point rating scale described above.

The way we talk

There are five behaviours to assess using the descriptions in the manual (below) and the six-point rating scale described above.

Conversational skills

There are eight behaviours in total to assess someone's conversational skills using the descriptions in the manual (below) and the six-point rating scale described above.

Assertiveness

There are eight behaviours to assess using the descriptions in the manual (below) and the six-point rating scale described above. Remember that assertiveness is the ability to express your thoughts and feelings in an appropriate and effective manner, not aggressively or passively or in a manner that adversely affects others. Therefore, if someone is 'always refusing' but is doing it in a way that is not appropriate or effective, you should consider how often they do it in a way that is 'appropriate to the context', and then you should rate them accordingly. So, if they never do it appropriately, they should be scored as a '1'. You may also consider how they appear to others. Do they come across as truly assertive? And if so, how often?

The f.4 scores then will generate the TASS wheel, which is viewed in s.4.

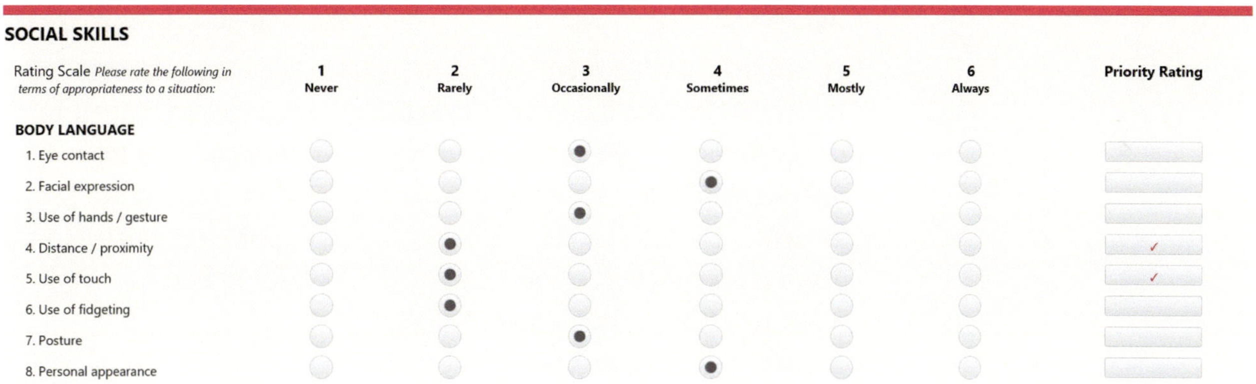

SOCIAL SKILLS

Rating Scale *Please rate the following in terms of appropriateness to a situation:*	1 Never	2 Rarely	3 Occasionally	4 Sometimes	5 Mostly	6 Always	Priority Rating
BODY LANGUAGE							
1. Eye contact	○	○	●	○	○	○	
2. Facial expression	○	○	○	●	○	○	
3. Use of hands / gesture	○	○	●	○	○	○	
4. Distance / proximity	○	●	○	○	○	○	✓
5. Use of touch	○	●	○	○	○	○	✓
6. Use of fidgeting	○	●	○	○	○	○	
7. Posture	○	○	●	○	○	○	
8. Personal appearance	○	○	○	●	○	○	

Figure 2.4 *f.4 Image of first screen*

f.4: Guidelines for scoring … body language

There are eight behaviours in total to assess someone's body language: eye contact, facial expression, gesture, distance, touch, fidgeting, posture and personal appearance. Each behaviour is assessed on the six-point rating scale described earlier.

Table 2.9 Scoring f.4: Body language

f.4: SCORING BODY LANGUAGE (questions 1–8)			
Skill	**Target**	**Description**	**Summary**
1. Eye contact	Able to use appropriate eye contact	*Where should people look?* In most situations, we look within the triangle from the eyebrows to the nose. If we know people well, we can also look towards the mouth. *How much?* During a typical conversation, we look at the person we are talking to about 45–60% of the time and when we are listening, our eye contact increases to 70–80%. *There is an eye contact dance …* • we start conversations and glance towards the other person • when the conversation takes hold, we look away • as we come to the end of a particular point, we look back at them to check the impact • the listener has been watching and is now ready to take over as the speaker, so they in turn begin to speak, look away, and then return to check the impact of their words … *Factors that affect eye contact* are distance, topic of conversation, what we are trying to achieve, relationship with the person, and personality. Ref. Kelly, 2019 pp 35–44	✓ looks within the triangle ✓ makes eye contact more when listening ✓ makes eye contact to initiate a conversation ✓ uses eye contact to manage turn taking ✓ eye contact is appropriate to the situation/topic

f.4: SCORING BODY LANGUAGE (questions 1–8)			
Skill	**Target**	**Description**	**Summary**
2. Facial expression	Able to use appropriate facial expressions	Facial expression should provide a running commentary on what someone is thinking or feeling. So, if we are happy, we look happy. The facial expression also reflects what the other person is saying/feeling, so if the person we are talking to is sad, then we also look sad. The lips, forehead, nostrils and facial blushing all play a part in expressing feelings through facial expressions. For example, tightly closed lips can show a restraint of an emotion, usually negative, and disappearing lips is related to stress or distress. *Micro expressions* 'leak out' in a split second and reveal our true feelings before we are able to activate our muscles into a facial expression. People have no conscious control over these. Ref. Kelly, 2019 pp 44–50	✓ facial expression is in line with what someone is saying or thinking ✓ facial expression reflects what the other person is saying
3. Use of hands/ gesture	Able to use appropriate gestures	The hands are the most spontaneous and communicative part of our body. We use our hands to greet people, illustrate a point and generally to express our feelings. The hands will communicate a lot and will influence how we are perceived by others and also why the hands are responsible for so much emotional leakage. As well as being informative about the person speaking, any gesture used should be appropriate to the situation and to the context of the conversation. Ref. Kelly, 2019 pp 21–4	✓ gestures are appropriate to the situation ✓ gestures reflect what the other person is saying ✓ gestures are used to enhance what is being said and to help the listener understand

f.4: SCORING BODY LANGUAGE (questions 1–8)			
Skill	**Target**	**Description**	**Summary**
4. Distance/ proximity	Uses appropriate distance	Distance or proximity can be described according to four zones: *The intimate zone: 15–45 cm.* Only people who are emotionally close to us are permitted into this space so this would include lovers, spouse, parents, children and close friends *The personal zone: 46 cm–1.22 m.* This is the most important one for people to learn as it is our 'one arm length' rule which is the ideal one in the Western world for most personal interaction. We are able to shake hands at this length and are less likely to cause offence by invading someone's 'bubble' *The social zone: 1.22–3.6 m.* We stand at this distance from people we don't know. This may include tradesmen doing work in our house or the new employee at work *The public zone: over 3.6 m.* When we have to address a large group of people, this is considered to be an acceptable distance from the front row There are several factors that will affect the distance rule: culture, height and situation. Ref. Kelly, 2019, pp 30–2	✓ distance is appropriate to the situation ✓ distance is appropriate to the relationship ✓ use of distance is altered if necessary, e.g., if the other person back away slightly
5. Use of touch	Uses appropriate touch	The use of touch is primarily used in ritualised greetings, e.g., handshake, or to reach out to connect with someone emotionally. Where we touch the other person can indicate dominance (e.g., hand on shoulder) or intimacy (touching hands) or sexual attraction (touching lower back). The most neutral/safe place to touch someone is the elbow. Appropriate touch should reflect the relationship with the other person and the situation/context.	✓ touch is appropriate to the situation ✓ touch is appropriate to the relationship

f.4: SCORING BODY LANGUAGE (*questions 1–8*)			
Skill	***Target***	***Description***	***Summary***
6. Use of fidgeting	Uses an appropriate amount of fidgeting	Fidgeting is any movement primarily with the hands and we can divide them into: *Displacement activities.* The amount we use our hands to fidget can give information about anxiety and nervous energy – movements that we perform when we're experiencing inner conflict or frustration, for example, repeatedly picking up phone/train ticket and looking at it (although not really looking at it). Feet also fidget – they may tap or bounce or kick. This displacement of energy shows that we can't wait to leave, or we are losing patience. *Self-comfort gestures.* These are movements that are directed towards our own body – comfort gestures that can indicate discomfort or anxiety. *Sensory seeking activities.* These are movements that are related to a sensory difficulty or need and may require a referral to an Occupational Therapist. Appropriate amount of fidgeting would refer to what is acceptable in the situation and takes into account the impact it has on others. Ref. Kelly, 2019 pp 20–1	✓ fidgeting is appropriate to the situation ✓ use of fidgeting is not distracting to the other person or themselves

f.4: SCORING BODY LANGUAGE (questions 1–8)			
Skill	**Target**	**Description**	**Summary**
7. Posture	Able to use appropriate posture	Posture refers to the way we stand or sit and can demonstrate confidence, dominance, sexuality, defensiveness and insecurity. The most significant factors are: *Open versus closed.* We use closed body positioning to indicate negative emotions and open posture to appear more positive and open to others. *Tense versus relaxed.* We use rigid posture to indicate negative emotions and relaxed to indicate confidence and positive emotions. Our posture needs to be appropriate to the situation and will often mirror the other person to show positive attitude towards them. Ref. Kelly, 2019, pp 24–30	✓ posture is appropriate to the situation ✓ posture is appropriate to the relationship with the other person
8. Personal appearance	Able to maintain and adapt an appropriate personal appearance	The use of personal appearance affects how people relate to us, particularly in the first seven seconds of meeting someone. We should consider the appropriateness of clothes, hair, accessories as well as personal hygiene and the situation. Ref. Kelly, 2019, pp 15–17	✓ personal appearance is appropriate to the situation ✓ the person shows an awareness of the impact personal appearance has on the other person

f.4: Guidelines for scoring ... the way we talk

There are five behaviours to assess: volume, rate, clarity, intonation and fluency. Each behaviour is assessed on the six-point rating scale described earlier.

Table 2.10 *Scoring f.4: The way we talk*

f.4: SCORING THE WAY WE TALK (questions 9–13)			
Skill	**Target**	**Description**	**Summary**
9. Volume	Able to use and adapt their volume appropriately	Volume is mostly dependant on the context, so we recognise when we need to raise our volume over background noise to be heard or lower it when someone is trying to sleep. Volume also reflects our emotional state, so anger is often reflected in louder volume and boredom in lower volume. Ref. Kelly, 2019 p 53	✓ volume is appropriate to the situation ✓ volume is adjusted to reflect the needs of the listener ✓ volume is varied and reflects emotional state
10. Rate	Able to use and adapt their rate appropriately	Rate of speech is mostly dependant on the context, so we recognise when we need to increase our rate if we see someone is in a hurry to leave or slow our rate if we see that someone has not understood. Rate also reflects our emotional state, so anger is often reflected in a faster rate and boredom in slower rate. Ref. Kelly, 2019 p 53	✓ rate is appropriate to the situation ✓ rate is adjusted to reflect the needs of the listener ✓ rate is varied and reflects emotional state
11. Clarity	Able to use speech that is clear and easily understood	Clarity of speech is associated with confidence and is also affected by our use of all the other paralinguistic skills, so if we use low volume, fast rate and monotonous intonation, our clarity will be affected. Clarity is also dependant on the context, so we recognise when we need to improve our clarity, for example if we need to impress the other person or if we see that someone has not understood. Clarity also reflects our emotional state, so we are more likely to mumble if we are bored or depressed. Ref. Kelly, 2019 p 53	✓ clarity is appropriate to the situation ✓ clarity is adjusted to reflect the needs of the listener ✓ clarity reflects emotional state

f.4: SCORING THE WAY WE TALK (questions 9–13)			
Skill	**Target**	**Description**	**Summary**
12. Intonation	*Able to use and adapt their intonation appropriately*	*Intonation is the way in which we alter our pitch and stress. The intonation pattern not only helps to communicate emotion but also helps the listener know which words to pay attention to. Intonation where there are 'up contours' is linked to happiness, interest, surprise, but also fear. A flat intonation shows a lack of interest or boredom.* *We also change our intonation to indicate we are just about to finish speaking which helps with turn taking. Intonation is also used to stress words or parts of words to help signify which part you want the listener to pay attention to and affects the meaning of a sentence.* *Ref. Kelly, 2019 p 53*	*✓ intonation is appropriate to the situation* *✓ intonation is adjusted to reflect the needs of the listener* *✓ intonation reflects emotional state*
13. Fluency	*Able to speak fluently with appropriate hesitations*	*Fluency of speech is how we connect the words without too much silence, hesitations or use of fillers such as 'um' or 'er'. It is linked to apprehension so the more apprehensive we are, the less fluent we tend to be and silence is associated with discomfort and negative feelings.* *Fluency is also associated with confidence and is dependent on the context.* *Ref. Kelly, 2019 p 53*	*✓ fluency is appropriate to the situation* *✓ fluency reflects emotional state*

f.4: Guidelines for scoring … conversational skills

There are eight behaviours in total to assess someone's conversational skills: listening, starting a conversation, taking turns, asking questions, answering questions, relevance, repairing and ending a conversation. Each behaviour is assessed on the six-point rating scale described earlier.

Table 2.11 Scoring f.4: Conversational skills

f.4: SCORING CONVERSATIONAL SKILLS (questions 14–21)			
Skill	**Target**	**Description**	**Summary**
14. Listening	Able to demonstrate appropriate listening	Listening has two parts: the auditory process of hearing, and the process of converting spoken language into meaning. So, we hear, interpret, evaluate and respond to the message. We may listen to understand; to evaluate or pass judgement; to accept and appreciate someone's point of view; or to empathise and attend to someone's thoughts, beliefs and feelings. Listening includes three processes: attending, following and reflecting, and involves both nonverbal and verbal behaviours. *Attending*: we use a posture of involvement, eye contact and appropriate body movement. *Following:* we use door openers ('please go on'); minimal encouragers ('mmm'); questions ('did you like it?'); attentive silence. *Reflecting:* we use paraphrasing, reflecting feelings, reflecting meanings and summative reflections. Ref. Kelly, 2019 pp 54–64	✓ attends appropriately within a conversation using good nonverbal behaviour ✓ uses appropriate verbal responses to demonstrate they are following the other person ✓ shows effective listening through reflecting what has been said

f.4: SCORING CONVERSATIONAL SKILLS (questions 14–21)			
Skill	*Target*	*Description*	*Summary*
15. *Starting a conversation*	Able to start a conversation appropriately	Starting a conversation is very dependent on the context of the interaction and what we want to achieve. There are two things to look out for when assessing this: Establish rapport: look for a relaxed and open body language, open facial expression and good eye contact. Opening line: this is dependent on whether we know the person but generally these should be personal but not too intrusive, authentic and adapted to the situation/person. Door openers: these can also be used to start a conversation in a less direct way, by using a statement, e.g., 'you look a bit fed up' or 'do you want to talk about it?', or silence and attending, e.g., eye contact and a posture of involvement to encourage someone to talk. Ref. Kelly, 2019 pp 67–73	✓ uses appropriate body language to start the conversation ✓ uses a variety of conversation starters that are appropriate to the context ✓ can use door openers when appropriate
16. *Taking turns*	Able to take turns appropriately	Turn taking is the ability to manage the relationship between speaker and listener within a conversation. There are several stages to it: The speaker has the floor: mostly this is one person, but they should keep an eye on how much they are talking, too little we are seen as uninterested or uncooperative; too much or for too long, and we are seen as boring and self-centred. Ending signals: the speaker sends ending signals such as lowering pitch and volume. Selecting the speaker: the speaker then looks at the next person and finishes with a steady gaze or selects them by name. The other person accepts the turn to speak: the other person returns the eye contact and starts speaking immediately. Using an opener: this might be a minimal response 'mmm, OK …', or express surprise or agreement 'yes!' or 'wow', or disagreement 'yes, but …' or changing the topic 'anyway …' Ref. Kelly, 2019 pp 81–6	✓ can talk for appropriate length of time within a conversation ✓ uses appropriate nonverbal signals to hand the conversation over to the other person ✓ uses appropriate responses or openers when starting their turn

f.4: SCORING CONVERSATIONAL SKILLS (questions 14–21)			
Skill	***Target***	***Description***	***Summary***
17. *Asking questions*	*Able to ask questions appropriately*	*Questions are an essential part of a conversation and should be accompanied by appropriate nonverbal signals and paralinguistic cues. Questions can be used to:* *Control the conversation: we use questions to focus on what we want to talk about.* *Set the mood: we use questions to affect someone's emotional state.* *Focus the discussion: we can use questions to speed up the discussion or get it back on track.* *Persuading others: we can ask questions about something we want the other person to consider.* *Open questions are more useful in conversations to get to know the other person.* *Ref. Kelly, 2019, pp 86–91*	*✓ can use appropriate types of questions within a conversation* *✓ uses appropriate nonverbal signals such as raised intonation, facial expression* *✓ uses open questions to encourage the listener*
18. *Answering questions*	*Able to answer questions appropriately*	*Answering a question appropriately will be dependent on the context, e.g., interview versus a quick chat by the coffee machine. If the answer is too short, we are seen as unfriendly or uncooperative, if they are too long, we are annoying or self-centred. Answering questions is usually an opportunity for self-disclosure and this happens in four ways:* *Observations/factual: telling people what we have done or experienced. These are used often when we meet people for the first time.* *Thoughts: revealing our judgements about what we have experienced.* *Feelings: how we feel or felt about something.* *Needs: telling people what we need or want.* *It is important to get the timing right when self-disclosing and to consider if the other person is in the right frame of mind to hear our disclosure; or if the disclosure fits the purpose of the conversation; or if the context or situation is appropriate.* *Ref. Kelly, 2019, pp 91–2*	*✓ can answer questions within a conversation using the right amount of information/length of reply* *✓ uses appropriate self-disclosure within a conversation* *✓ shows an awareness of the other person and situation when answering questions*

f.4: SCORING CONVERSATIONAL SKILLS (questions 14–21)			
Skill	**Target**	**Description**	**Summary**
19. Relevance	*Can maintain, develop and change topics appropriately*	*Relevance means saying things that are pertinent to the discussion or conversation. However, this is relative and very dependent on the context and can be seen as being 'in the eye of the beholder'. However, as a rule, a relevant remark usually responds to something said in the speaker's last sentence and is related to the purpose of the conversational goal. We are showing our attentiveness by staying on topic. If we want to change the topic, we need to do this subtly:* *wait for the person to finish speaking* *wait for a longer-than-normal pause* *try to 'wrap up' a topic and then pause* *use one of the following 'soooo …' or 'ANYway …' 'before I forget …'* *Ref. Kelly, 2019, pp 93–5*	*✓ uses relevant remarks within a conversation* *✓ can stay on topic when appropriate to do so* *✓ shows an awareness of how to change topic using nonverbal and verbal markers*
20. Repairing a breakdown	*Able to maintain relevance by repairing appropriately*	*When a breakdown occurs in a conversation, there are several ways in which we can repair whilst taking our turn. For example:* *Correcting a mistake: something has been misunderstood or misheard and we need to correct it quickly.* *Adding more information: if someone is confused by our answer and we need to provide more.* *Telling them something they already know: this is not always a problem, unless it is something we should know they know. We need to quickly apologise to repair this.* *Going on for too long: if the other person begins to look distracted or uncomfortable, we need to apologise and give them a chance to speak.* *Ref. Kelly, 2019, pp 92–3*	*✓ able to correct mistakes within a conversation* *✓ can add more information when needed* *✓ shows an awareness of when they need to stop and hand the conversation over to the other person*

f.4: SCORING CONVERSATIONAL SKILLS (*questions 14–21*)			
Skill	***Target***	***Description***	***Summary***
21. *Ending a conversation*	*Able to end a conversation appropriately*	*Ending a conversation involves a sequence of actions but is dependent on the reason why we need to end the conversation.* *There are four main types of closure:* *Factual: summarise what has been said, check we have understood '… is that OK?', or state a future plan 'I'll see you tomorrow'.* *Motivational: when we want to encourage someone in something with a statement that is motivating or thought-provoking, or an idea for the future.* *Social: to show that we have enjoyed the conversation but either commenting on what we have been talking about 'that's been helpful – thank you', or a more general personal comment 'it's been lovely talking to you'.* *Perceptual: using physical movement or positionings e.g., shifting body posture, breaking eye contact, and verbal markers e.g., 'anyway …', to indicate that we need to end the conversation.* *Ref. Kelly, 2019 pp 73–8*	✓ *uses appropriate body language to end the conversation* ✓ *uses appropriate verbal cues to indicate the end of the conversation* ✓ *uses a variety of ways to end the conversation that are appropriate to the context*

f.4: Guidelines for scoring … assertiveness

There are eight situations in which assertive behaviour is appropriate and which are assessed: expressing feelings, standing up for yourself, making suggestions, refusing, disagreeing, complaining, apologising and requesting explanations. Each behaviour is assessed on the six-point rating scale described earlier.

Table 2.12 Scoring f.4: Assertiveness

f.4: SCORING ASSERTIVENESS (questions 22–9)			
Skill	**Target**	**Description**	**Summary**
22. Expressing feelings	Able to express their feelings appropriately	Expressing feelings comes into many of the assertive responses and situations and so is the first area to teach in assertiveness. The first step in expressing feelings assertively is to understand what we are feeling. We do this in three ways: Listen to our emotions: take note of how we are feeling. Listen to our body: take note of what is happening in our body. Express the feeling: the more we express our emotions, the more we sharpen our emotional awareness. Expressing our feelings assertively involves four steps: name the emotion: 'I feel angry' explain and describe: 'I am feeling … because …' use supporting body language: our facial expression and posture should mirror the emotion use supporting paralinguistic skills: using a clear, calm, measured speech will help people listen to us Ref. Kelly, 2019 pp 108–10	✓ can express and describe their feelings appropriately within a conversation ✓ uses clear messages such as 'I am feeling … because …' ✓ uses appropriate body language to support their message ✓ uses appropriate paralinguistic skills to support their message

f.4: SCORING ASSERTIVENESS (questions 22–9)			
Skill	**Target**	**Description**	**Summary**
23. *Standing up for self or beliefs*	*Able to stand up for themselves appropriately*	*Standing up for ourselves involves telling people how we feel and what we think but also what we believe in and defending our point of view. It is important to consider:* *The other person: what are their thoughts and feelings? Can we imagine what is going on for them? Could we simply ask them?* *Our own point of view: how much do we need to justify or explain ourselves? Sometimes it is OK to accept that opinions differ. Consider how we can clarify our opinion without appearing defensive or attacking them.* *stop and think – do we agree with what is being said or done? Do we need to say something?* *use assertive body language to show we are confident in what we think* *use a calm voice and speak clearly.* *We can try saying 'I think … because …'* *Ref. Kelly, 2019 p 110*	*✓ can tell the other person what they think or believe in appropriately within a conversation* *✓ uses clear messages such as 'I think … because …'* *✓ uses appropriate body language to support their message and to appear confident* *✓ uses appropriate paralinguistic skills to support their message*
24. *Making suggestions or giving opinions*	*Able to make suggestions or give opinions appropriately*	*Making suggestions involves being able to give our ideas and opinions in a way that is heard and listened to. At a simple level it may be a suggestion to help someone out or help solve a problem or it may be a suggestion that centres around an emotion. The context is important as always, but it is important to remember to listen to their response and to respond accordingly. So, the rules are:* *wait for a pause – then we can give our idea or arrange a time to talk to someone* *use a calm voice and speak clearly.* *We can try saying 'I think that …' or 'maybe we could …'* *listen to the other person and respond appropriately* *Ref. Kelly, 2019 p 111*	*✓ can make suggestions appropriately within a conversation* *✓ uses clear messages such as 'I think that …'* *✓ uses appropriate nonverbal skills to support their message* *✓ listens to the other person and responds accordingly*

f.4: SCORING ASSERTIVENESS (questions 22–9)			
Skill	***Target***	**Description**	***Summary***
25. *Refusing with reason/ apology*	*Able to refuse appropriately*	*Refusing assertively is one of the more difficult assertive skills. There are different ways to say no and the context here is essential to choosing the right way.* *Reflective listening and then 'no': reflect on the content of a reasonable request and then say 'no'.* *The reasoned 'no': we say no and give a reason that is sincere.* *The rain check 'no': we say no to a request but immediately suggest an alternative.* *The broken record 'no': when someone is repeatedly asking us something and won't take no for an answer. We use a one-sentence refusal statement several times.* *The flat-out 'no': we use this when the request is not reasonable. We say no but offer no reason or rain check.* *So, the rules for refusing are:* *stop and think – do we agree with what is being asked? Do we have a choice?* *use assertive body language to show confidence* *use a calm voice and speak clearly* *say 'no' and then if appropriate give a reason or apology* *Ref. Kelly, 2019 pp 111–12*	*✓ can say no appropriately within a conversation* *✓ uses clear messages and gives a reason or an apology if necessary* *✓ uses appropriate body language to support their message* *✓ uses appropriate paralinguistic skills to support their message*

f.4: SCORING ASSERTIVENESS (questions 22–9)			
Skill	**Target**	**Description**	**Summary**
26. Disagreeing with reason or compromise	*Able to disagree appropriately*	*The skill of disagreeing is important so that other people understand how we think and feel. We may want to express our opinions, or we may have a better idea, or a compromise that will make others happy as well as us.* *The rules for disagreeing are:* *stop and think – do we agree with what is being said or suggested?* *remember to listen and respect the other person's opinion. Is there a compromise?* *use a calm voice and speak clearly and remember to use assertive body language* *try saying 'I'm sorry I disagree …' or 'maybe we should …'* *Ref. Kelly, 2019 pp 112–13*	*✓ can disagree appropriately within a conversation* *✓ uses clear messages and gives a reason or a compromise if necessary* *✓ uses appropriate nonverbal skills to support their message* *✓ listens to the other person and responds accordingly*
27. Complaining with reason	*Able to complain appropriately*	*It is important to complain when we feel something is not right or when we have been misled or sold something faulty. Some things we can do to help ensure we complain appropriately are to consider beforehand what we hope to gain from complaining; who is the right person to talk to; get our emotions under control first; consider a 'complaint sandwich'; and admit our part of the problem if appropriate.* *The rules for complaining are:* *stop and think – who should we talk to? What are our rights?* *remember to use assertive body language and to show we are confident in what we say* *use a calm voice and speak clearly explain why we are not happy. Try saying 'I'm not happy … because …'* *Ref. Kelly, 2019 pp 113–14*	*✓ can complain appropriately* *✓ uses clear messages and gives a reason for the complaint* *✓ uses appropriate nonverbal skills to support their message* *✓ listens to the other person and responds accordingly*

f.4: SCORING ASSERTIVENESS (questions 22–9)			
Skill	**Target**	**Description**	**Summary**
28. Apologising shows remorse/ responsibility	*Able to apologise appropriately*	*Apologising is important if we have made a mistake or upset someone and it should ideally be done quickly and with meaning so that people know it is genuine. The way we say sorry is dependent on the severity of the situation and how much we need to apologise. There are four steps to saying sorry:* *Express remorse: start with the words 'I'm sorry …'* *Admit responsibility: for our actions or behaviour and acknowledge what we did 'I was wrong to …'* *Make amends: take action that is proportionate to make the situation right* *Promise it won't happen again: we should reassure the other person that it won't happen again 'From now on …'* *The rules are:* *stop and think – who should we apologise to? Does it need to be a big or little sorry?* *remember to use assertive body language and to show them we mean what we are saying* *use a sincere tone of voice and express regret* *take responsibility. Try saying 'I'm sorry … that was my fault …' and if appropriate do something to make up for it* *Ref. Kelly, 2019 pp 114–15*	*✓ can say sorry when it is appropriate* *✓ uses clear messages and admits responsibility* *✓ uses appropriate nonverbal skills to support their message* *✓ offers to remedy the situation with an appropriate action*

f.4: SCORING ASSERTIVENESS (questions 22–9)			
Skill	**Target**	**Description**	**Summary**
29. Requesting explanations	*Requests explanations appropriately*	*Requesting explanations is important if we don't understand something or we feel we need more information. It is important to do this clearly so that other people can understand what we need and can give us the right explanation.* *The rules for requesting explanations are:* *stop and think – do we understand what has been said or asked of us?* *use a calm voice, speak clearly and remember to use assertive body language* *ask a question or for an explanation* *say 'I am sorry I don't understand, could you explain?'* *remember to say thank you* *Ref. Kelly, 2019 p 115*	✓ *can ask for explanations if necessary* ✓ *uses clear messages and asks an appropriate question* ✓ *uses appropriate nonverbal skills to support their message* ✓ *says thank you*

f.4: Guidelines for analysing

In summary, the assessor is reviewing the areas of the wheel and the ratings within each area. Simply put, the more the wheel is filled in, the more of a strength that area is for that person.

The assessor would expect to see the hierarchy reflected in the wheel, so generally, nonverbal behaviours are stronger than verbal behaviours, and both are stronger than assertiveness. If the assessment shows you that the assertiveness section or the conversation skills section are stronger than the body language and the way we talk sections, it is worth going back and checking your ratings.

It may be possible that the information you have gained from others is inaccurate. For example, have they misunderstood what you mean by 'assertiveness' and have described behaviour that is aggressive or arrogant?

In each section, look at how many of the behaviours have different ratings. In short,

- *ratings of 5 and 6 in all behaviours would indicate a clear strength in this area*
- *ratings of 1–4 in all behaviours would indicate a clear need to work on this area*
- *if there is a majority of 1–4 ratings but a couple of strengths, then this indicates that it is still important to work on this area*
- *if there is a majority of 5 and 6 ratings, but a couple of needs, then it is important to look at the behaviours that have been rated 1–4 and consider if they are essential to work on before you can move to the next section, or whether you can move onto the next section*
- *you will also need to consider the person's motivations and quality of life to help guide your intervention (see section on social validity and motivation in the introduction)*

Below is a summary of how to analyse the results of each section.

Table 2.13 *Analysing f.4*

f.4: ANALYSING THE TASS	
Section	**Where does this guide me?**
All sections	The hierarchy of skills should be referred to for all sections: 1. self-awareness and self-esteem 2. body language 3. the way we talk 4. conversations 5. assertiveness
Body language	• remember that nonverbal behaviours should be worked on prior to verbal and assertive behaviours but after self-awareness and self-esteem (if this has been assessed to be an area of need in f.2) • difficulties in this area will be impacting on conversational and assertiveness skills so body language is taught first • depending on the age of the person you could use the following resources: ○ *Talkabout for Children: developing social skills* (Level 1 Talkabout Body Language) ○ *Talkabout 2nd edition* (Level 1 Talkabout Body Language) ○ *Talkabout for Teenagers* (Level 2 Talkabout Body Language) • strengths in this area would indicate that you are able to prioritise work on the way they talk or their verbal or assertiveness skills
The way we talk	• remember that nonverbal behaviours (the way we talk is a nonverbal behaviour) should be worked on prior to verbal and assertive behaviours but after self-awareness and self-esteem and body language if these are areas of need • difficulties in this area will be impacting on conversational and assertiveness skills so are taught first • depending on the age of the person you could use the following resources: ○ *Talkabout for Children: developing social skills* (Level 2 Talkabout Talking, Topic 2: Talkabout Speaking) ○ *Talkabout 2nd edition* (Level 2 Talkabout the Way We Talk) ○ *Talkabout for Teenagers* (Level 3 Talkabout Talking, Topic 1) • strengths in this area would indicate that you are able to prioritise work on verbal or assertiveness skills

f.4: ANALYSING THE TASS	
Section	***Where does this guide me?***
Conversational skills	• *remember that verbal behaviours should be worked on prior to assertive behaviours but after self-awareness and self-esteem, body language and the way we talk if these are areas of need* • *difficulties in this area will be impacting on assertiveness skills so are taught first* • *depending on the age of the person you could use the following resources:* ○ *Talkabout for Children: developing social skills* (Level 2 Talkabout Talking) ○ *Talkabout 2nd edition* (Level 3 Talkabout Conversations) ○ *Talkabout for Teenagers* (Level 3 Talkabout Talking) • *strengths in this area would indicate that you are able to prioritise work on assertiveness skills*
Assertiveness	• Remember that assertive behaviours should be worked on last and only when the person has enough strengths in all the other areas assessed: self-awareness and self-esteem, body language, the way we talk and conversations. • Depending on the age of the person you could use the following resources: ○ *Talkabout for Children: developing social skills* (Level 3 Talkabout Assertiveness) ○ *Talkabout 2nd edition* (Level 4 Talkabout Assertiveness) ○ Talkabout for Teenagers (Level 5 Talkabout Assertiveness) • Strengths in this area would indicate that you are able to consider work on friendship or relationship skills or no further intervention is needed.
Priority rating	• Are there any priorities highlighted in an area where it would be clinically appropriate to start intervention, considering the hierarchy of social skills? If so, these should be prioritised first. • If the person has highlighted priority areas in a clinical area where it is not appropriate to start work, can they be supported to understand how planned intervention targets will help the person to reach their long-term goal? This might include, for example, an explanation of the hierarchy of social skills.

Summary charts

Summary charts

In this section, you can view the summary information from all parts of the assessment.

s.1 Associated factors *and* **quality of life**. *This is a summary bar chart for both associated factors and quality of life, generated from f.1 (initial information).*

s.2 Interview summary. *This is a summary bar chart for the client interview generated from the ratings at the end of f.2.*

s.3 Self-rating summary. *This is a summary bar chart for the self-rating scale generated from f.3.*

s.4 TASS wheel. *This is the TASS wheel which summarises the person's social skills profile and is generated from f.4.*

s.5 Areas of high priority. *This is a summary of all areas of high priority which have been generated from all sections of the assessments (f.1–4).*

Analysing the summary charts

s.1 Associated factors and quality of life

This is the summary of all quantitative information collated on associated factors and quality of life within f.1 – initial information.

This is presented as two bar charts and will form part of your baseline assessment. Associated factors are important to measure, as the presence of these may hinder or help intervention. The quality of life indicators may also be linked to social communication needs and the potential long-term effects of intervention.

With this in mind, you may want to reassess these factors at a later date to report on the impact of intervention.

Associated factors

If there are areas of need in this chart, consider if any require liaison with other professionals e.g., teaching staff. Would 1:1 strategies with regards to behaviour be beneficial (e.g., comic strip, conversations problem solving, Social Stories™) or is a behaviour support plan required?

Quality of life

If there are areas of need in this chart, consider how intervention targets can link to improving quality of life for the person (see hierarchy). Are any of these areas a long-term goal of intervention? Do any other professionals need to be involved?

s.2 Self-awareness and self-esteem interview

This is the summary of f.2 – the interview. f.2 is scored using seven self-awareness and self-esteem targets and these form a baseline score for any intervention and are shown as a bar chart.

Challenges in this area: You will want to consider whether your assessment suggests low self-awareness and self-esteem. This would indicate that this is where intervention may need to start as this will impact on social communication. People with low self-esteem may also have challenges in coping with their emotions so make sure work on emotions is included into your self-awareness and self-esteem work.

Depending on the age of the person you could look at the following resources:

- *Talkabout for Children: developing self-awareness and self-esteem*
- *Talkabout for Teenagers* (level 1)
- *Talkabout for Adults*

Deciding to work on self-awareness and self-esteem: If you are going to work on this area, you can now use the baseline scores to measure the impact of intervention. We would recommend using a simple spreadsheet to show progress from the baseline scores to mid-term scores to end of intervention, and then to demonstrate this in a bar chart. The authors are happy to share the spreadsheets they have devised to do this with you if this would be helpful. Please contact the publishers.

Strengths in this area: Strengths in this area would indicate that you are able to prioritise work on their social skills.

s.3 Self-rating scale

This is the summary of f.3 – the self-rating scale. This includes ratings related to self-awareness and self-esteem, several social skills and a few associated and quality of life factors. This form will only have been completed if you considered it was appropriate for the person.

Guidelines for analysing

The self-rating scale can add a wealth of information to the holistic assessment of a person's social skills profile and will also help to inform your intervention plan.

Some points to consider when analysing the results would be:

- Are there some potential areas of need for the person, i.e., which areas did they rate as most difficult?
- Does the person either rate themselves to be consistently low or consistently high and what might the reasons for this be?
- Where any needs are highlighted, are these in the same area of the hierarchy? For example, does a person find all areas of self-esteem very difficult?
- How do the person's ratings compare to other parts of the assessment, i.e., the assessor's ratings in the interview and TASS? Where are the areas of agreement or discrepancy and what might be the reasons for this?

- *Based on the person's own judgements compared to others in forms 2 and 4, what would be the assessor's view of the person's self-awareness? Does the assessor need to carry out some observations to determine this?*
- *Which areas does the person view as the most important? Are these the same as the areas of need, or are they different?*
- *How do the importance ratings compare to the priority ratings in forms 1, 2 and 4? Does everyone agree about the areas of priority and therefore should intervention start here? If there are areas of disagreement, why is this? Is the person demonstrating low self-awareness and therefore should intervention start here? Is more information needed about how they present in different environments?*
- *What are the top priorities for this person, and based on the rest of the assessment is this an appropriate place to start intervention?*

s.4 The TASS wheel

This is the summary of f.4 – the Talkabout Assessment of Social Skills (TASS). The wheel summarises each section in a different colour: body language (red), the way we talk (blue), conversational skills (green) and assertiveness (yellow). You are reviewing the ratings within each area and the more the wheel is filled in, the more of a strength that area is for that person. In particular, look out for the following:

The hierarchy: *You would expect to see the hierarchy reflected in the wheel, so generally, nonverbal behaviours (body language and the way we talk) are stronger than verbal behaviours (conversational skills), and both are stronger than assertiveness.*

1. *body language*
2. *the way we talk*
3. *conversations*
4. *assertiveness*

The number of strengths and challenges in each area:

In each section, look at how many of the behaviours have different ratings. In short,

- *ratings of 5 and 6 in all behaviours would indicate a clear strength in this area*
- *ratings of 1–4 in all behaviours would indicate a clear need to work on this area*
- *if there is a majority of 1–4 ratings but a couple of strengths, then this indicates that it is still important to work on this area*
- *if there is a majority of 5 and 6 ratings, but a couple of needs, then it is important to look at the behaviours that have been rated 1–4 and consider if they are essential to work on before you can move to the next section, or whether you can move onto the next section*
- *you will also need to consider the person's motivations and quality of life to help guide your intervention (see section on social validity and motivation)*

Deciding to work on social skills: *If you are going to work on any of these four areas of social skills, the authors recommend that you use a simple spreadsheet to evidence the impact of intervention.*

Use the baseline scores from the TASS and then when you have reassessment scores, you can create bar charts to evidence progress.

s.5 Priority ratings

This is the summary of all behaviours and factors that have been highlighted as an area of high priority across all assessment forms f.1–4. A priority rating is included in all the forms. This is to provide an indication of how important each area is to the person, and if they are having a significant impact on the person's social communication. Some of these areas may not be attended to directly via a social skills intervention and may require the involvement of other professionals. However, it is still important to assess the priorities pre- and post-intervention, to ensure intervention is socially valid and to assess if intervention has had a direct or indirect impact on any of the areas highlighted.

These are listed accordingly under the headings: associated factors and quality of life, self-awareness and self-esteem, self-rating scale and social skills (TASS).

Guidelines for analysing

- is there some similarity between, or repetition of, areas highlighted as priorities?
- are there priorities highlighted in an area where it would be clinically appropriate to start intervention, considering the hierarchy of social skills?
- if the person has highlighted priority areas in the self-rating scale in a clinical area where it is not appropriate to start work, can they be supported to understand how intervention targets will help the person to reach their long-term goal?

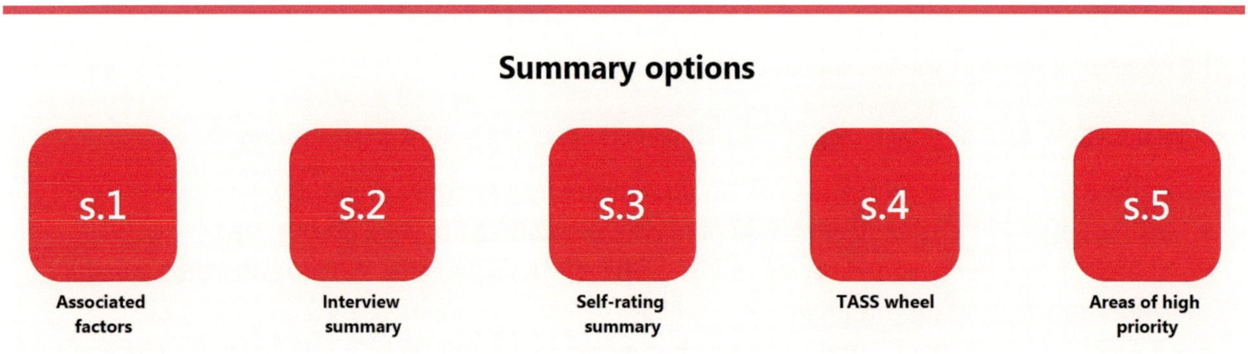
Summary options
s.1
Associated factors
s.2
Interview summary
s.3
Self-rating summary
s.4
TASS wheel
s.5
Areas of high priority

Figure 2.5 Image of summary options

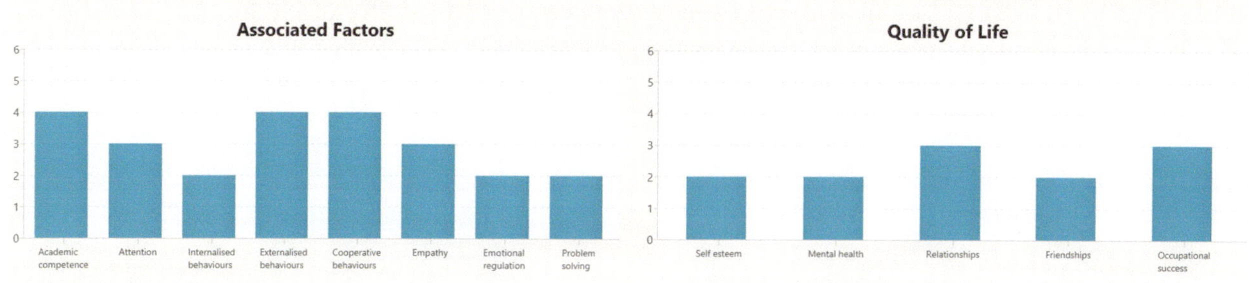

Figure 2.6 Image of s.1

This is the summary of all quantitative information collated on associated factors and quality of life within f.1 – initial information.

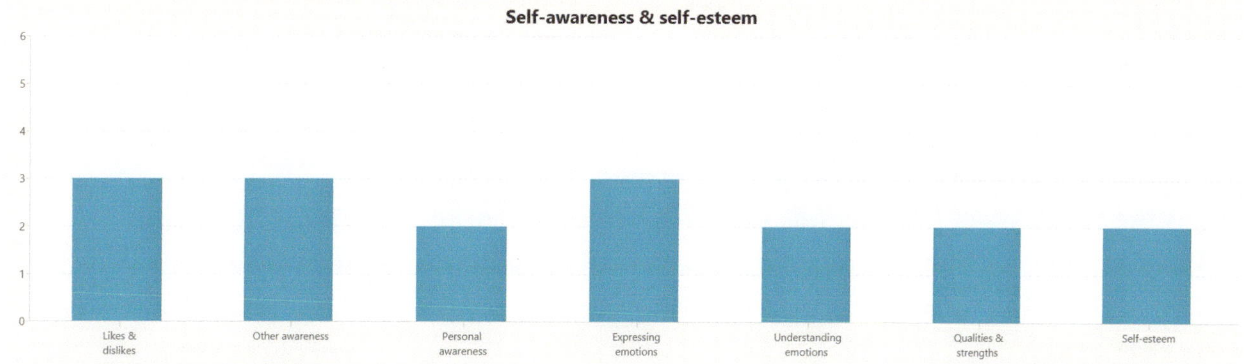

Figure 2.7 Image of s.2

This is the summary of f.2 – the interview. f.2 is scored using seven self-awareness and self-esteem targets and these form a baseline score for any intervention and are shown as a bar chart.

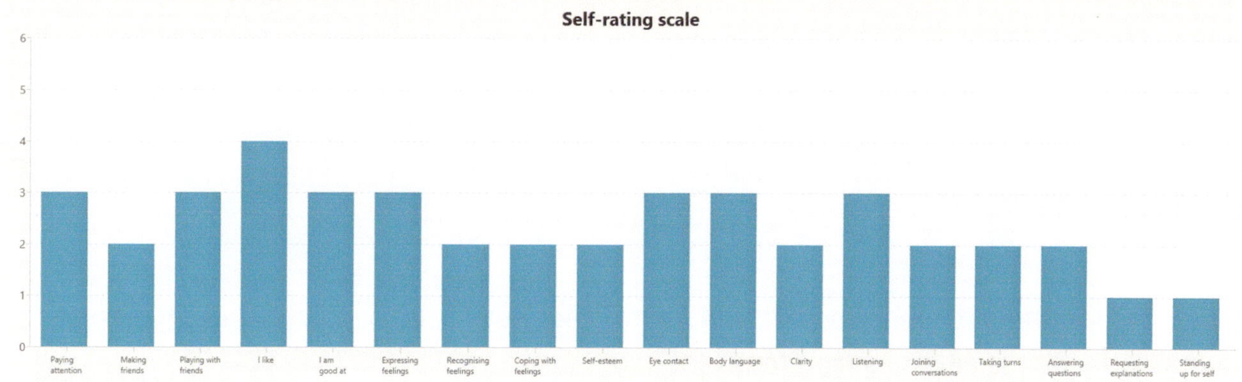

Figure 2.8 Image of s.3

This is the summary of f.3 – the self-rating scale. This includes ratings related to self-awareness and self-esteem, several social skills and a few associated and quality of life factors. This bar chart will only be present if f.3 has been completed (i.e., you considered it was appropriate for the person).

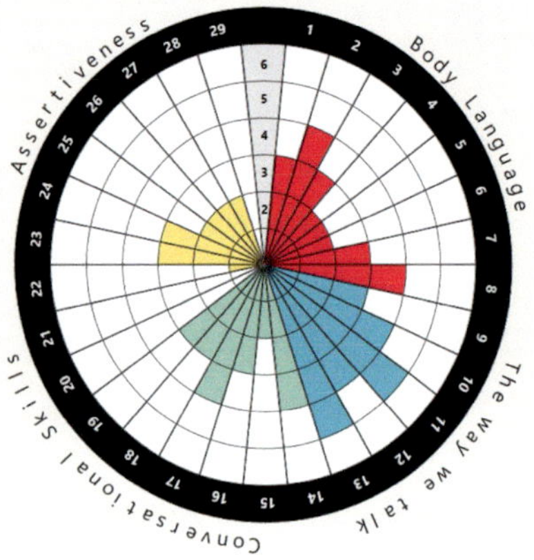

BODY LANGUAGE	THE WAY WE TALK	CONVERSATIONAL SKILLS	ASSERTIVENESS
1. Eye contact	9. Volume	14. Listening	22. Expressing feelings
2. Facial expression	10. Rate	15. Starting a conversation	23. Standing up for self
3. Gesture	11. Clarity	16. Taking turns	24. Making suggestions
4. Distance	12. Intonation	17. Asking questions	25. Refusing
5. Touch	13. Fluency	18. Answering questions	26. Disagreeing
6. Fidgeting		19. Relevance	27. Complaining
7. Posture		20. Repairing	28. Apologising
8. Personal appearance		21. Ending a conversation	29. Requesting explainations

Figure 2.9 *Image of s.4*

This is the summary of f.4 – the Talkabout Assessment of Social Skills (TASS). The wheel summarises each section in a different colour: body language (red), the way we talk (blue), conversational skills (green) and assertiveness (yellow).

The following have been marked as high priority

Associated and quality of life factors	Self-awareness and self-esteem	Self-Rating Scale	Social Skills (TASS)
3 Internalised behaviours 7 Emotional regulation 9 Self esteem 12 Friendships	3 Personal awareness 4 Expressing emotions 5 Understanding emotions 7 Self-esteem	2 Making friends 8 Coping with my feelings 9 Feeling good about being me 14 Joining in conversations 18 Standing up for myself	4 Distance 5 Touch

Figure 2.10 *Image of s.5*

This is the summary of all behaviours and factors that have been highlighted as an area of high priority across all assessment forms f.1–4.

References

CASEL. (2023). What Is the CASEL Framework? https://casel.org/fundamentals-of-sel/what-is-the-casel-framework/.

Clarke A., Sorgenfrei M., Mulcahy J., Davie P., Friedrich C., & McBride T. (2021). Adolescent Mental Health: A Systematic Review on the Effectiveness of School-Based Interventions. *Early Intervention Foundation*, July, 1–87.

Gresham F. (2015). Evidence-Based Social Skills Interventions for Students at Risk for EBD. *Remedial and Special Education, 36*(2), 100–104.

Gresham F., & Elliott S. (2008). *SSiS Social Skills Improvement System*. Bloomington, MN: NCS Pearson, Inc.

Kelly A. (1996). *TALKABOUT*. London: Speechmark.

Kelly A. (2013). *TALKABOUT for CHILDREN: Developing Friendship Skills*. London: Speechmark.

Kelly A. (2016). *TALKABOUT*, 2nd edition. London: Speechmark.

Kelly A. (2018*a*) *TALKABOUT for CHILDREN: Developing Self-Awareness and Self-Esteem*, 2nd edition. London: Speechmark.

Kelly A. (2018*b*) *TALKABOUT for CHILDREN: Developing Social Skills*, 2nd edition. London: Speechmark.

Kelly A. (2019). *Social Skills: Developing Effective Interpersonal Communication*. London: Speechmark.

Kelly A., & Sains B. (2009). *TALKABOUT for Teenagers*. London: Speechmark.

Kelly A., & Sains B. (2010). *TALKABOUT Assessment Tool*. London: Speechmark.

Kelly A., & Green A. (2014). *TALKABOUT for ADULTS: Developing Self-Awareness and Self-Esteem*. London: Speechmark.

Matson J. L., Matson M. L., & Rivet T. T. (2007). Social-Skills Treatments for Children with Autism an Overview. *Behavior Modification, 31*(5), 682–707.

Appendices

This section includes

Worked Example 1: Teenager

Worked Example 2: 9 year old

TASS assessment forms (blank)

Name: WORKED EXAMPLE: *Teenager* *DoB: 16 years old*

INITIAL INFORMATION	**FORM 1**
A. PERSONAL INFORMATION	
Address	*Lives with parents*
Telephone number	
School/occupation	*Home schooling*
Contact at school	
Contact at home	
B. DESCRIPTION OF PERSON'S SOCIAL SKILLS	
Reason for referral	*Help with social skills*
Relevant diagnoses	ASD
External factors which influence social skills (e.g., environmental, cultural, events)	Noise
Examples of situations the person finds difficult	1. *Meeting friends*
	2. *Family gatherings*
	3. *Meeting new people*

Name: *WORKED EXAMPLE: Teenager* DoB: *16 years old*

C. ASSOCIATED FACTORS							
Rating scale Please rate the following	1 Never	2 Rarely	3 Occasionally	4 Sometimes	5 Mostly	6 Always	Priority rating
1. Reaches expected academic goals						✓	
2. Demonstrates expected attention and listening skills					✓		
3. Manages internalised behaviours effectively *(e.g., anxiety)*	✓						✓
4. Manages externalised behaviours effectively *(e.g., aggression)*		✓					
5. Demonstrates cooperative behaviours *(e.g., sharing, following rules)*						✓	
6. Shows empathy	✓						
7. Able to regulate emotions	✓						✓
8. Able to problem solve		✓					
D. QUALITY OF LIFE							
1. Has healthy self-esteem		✓					
2. Has good mental health	✓						✓
3. Develops and maintains close relationships *(e.g., family, romantic)*		✓					✓
4. Develops and maintains friendships		✓					✓
5. Achieves occupational success *(e.g., school, higher ed., paid/unpaid employment)*					✓		

Name: WORKED EXAMPLE: *Teenager*

DoB: *16 years old*

E. ACTION PLAN	
Long-term goal *Please describe what the person would like to achieve as a result of intervention.*	*To gain confidence in social situations.* *Work towards making and keeping friends.* *Aim for better emotional regulation* *To be able to return to educational setting*
Any other comments	
Next steps	*Social skills group*
Person(s) completing form	*Mother*
Date	*January 2022*

Name: WORKED EXAMPLE: Teenager DoB: 16 years old

SELF-AWARENESS AND SELF-ESTEEM INTERVIEW		**FORM 2**
1. Let's talk about some of the things you like doing. *Can you tell me three things you like or enjoy?* *Example prompts: favourite lesson; favourite game; hobbies or activities*	**Verbal Prompt?** √	**Visual Prompt?** √
1. Guitar 2. Hockey 3. Statistics or maths	1. 2. 3.	1. 2. 3.
2. Is there anything you really don't like doing? *Can you think of three things you don't like or don't enjoy?* *Example prompts: lesson; game; hobbies or activities*		
1. Running 2. Playing violin 3. Spinach	1. 2. 3.	1. 2. 3.
3. Let's talk about someone you know. Do you have a good friend? Or a teacher you like? *Can you tell me three things about them?* *Example prompts: what they look like; why you like them; what kind of person are they?*		
1. She is funny 2. She is always dyeing her hair 3. She's tall	1. 2. 3.	1. 2. 3.
4. What do you think that person would say about you? *Can you think of two things that they would say about you?* *Example prompts: what you look like; why they like you; what kind of person you are?*		
1. Self-conscious 2. Can be difficult to read/emotionally shy	1. 2.	1. 2.

Name: WORKED EXAMPLE: Teenager DoB: 16 years old

5. Let's talk about the way you look. *Can you tell me three things about the way you look?* *Example prompts: hair colour/length; height, eye colour; skin; clothing; you can use visual prompt 1*	**Verbal Prompt?** √	**Visual Prompt?** √
1. Short hair	1.	1.
2. Quite short	2.	2.
3. Often wear dark colours	3.	3.
6. How are you feeling today? *Using the feelings board, can you tell me how you are feeling and why?* *Example prompts: are you happy; sad; worried or something else? use visual prompt 2 (feelings)*		
1. Alright, bit anxious. Neutral. Worried	1.	1. Feelings board ✓
7. Let's talk about your feelings more … *Can you think of something that makes you feel … happy? excited? sad? angry? worried?* *Example prompts: subjects at school; activities or hobbies*		
1. Happy or excited? Doing something with my friends – coffee and a chat but I'm scared of awkward silences	1.	1.
2. Sad, angry or worried? Family arguments, one of my friends not feeling great	2.	2.
8. What helps you when you are feeling sad, or angry or worried? *Can you think of anything that helps you?* *Example prompts: an activity or a person*		
1. Noise-cancelling headphones	1.	1.
2. Music, Lego	2.	2.

Name: WORKED EXAMPLE: *Teenager* DoB: *16 years old*

9. What are you good at? *Can you think of two things that you are good at?* *Example prompts: subjects at school; activities or hobbies*	**Verbal Prompt?** √	**Visual Prompt?** √
1. *Maths* 2. *Giving advice on emotional stuff*	1. 2.	1. 2.
10. Is there anything that you find difficult? *Is there something that you find hard at school or home?* *Example prompts: subjects at school; activities or hobbies*		
1. *Having no structure if I'm meeting a friend* 2. *Not being prepared for things/don't know what is happening*	1. 2.	1. 2.
11. What kind of person do you think you are? *Can you think of three words to describe what you are like?* *Example prompts: chatty or quiet; hard-working or lazy; you can use visual prompt 3*		
1. *Sensitive* 2. *Academic* 3. *Emotional*	1. 2. 3.	1. 2. 3.
12. Tell me the best thing about being you. *Is there 1 thing you really like about being you?* *Example prompts: about themselves/their family; school; activities*		
1. *My life is a bit different to other teenagers but home schooling is cool*	1.	1.
13. If you could change one thing about being you, what would it be? *Example prompts: about themselves/their family; school; activities*		
1. *Emotional difficulties – would be easier without them*	1.	1.
14. Is there anything you would like to ask me? *I've asked you lots of questions, so is there anything you would like to ask me?*		
1. *Don't think so*	1.	1.

Name: WORKED EXAMPLE: *Teenager*

DoB: 16 *years old*

SELF-AWARENESS AND SELF-ESTEEM SUMMARY							**FORM 2**
Rating scale	1 **No, never** *even with lots of support*	2 **Yes, but *rarely*** *and only with lots of support*	3 **Yes, occasionally** *or with some support*	4 **Yes, sometimes** *or in familiar situations only*	5 **Yes, mostly** *but not always*	6 **Yes, *always***	*Priority rating*
SELF/OTHER AWARENESS							
1. Likes and dislikes: *is able to describe three things they like and three things they dislike (Qu 1 & 2)*					✓		
2. Other awareness: *is able to describe someone else using at least three descriptive words (Qu 3)*					✓		
3. Personal awareness: *is able to describe the way they look using at least three descriptive words (Qu 5)*					✓		
EMOTIONS							
4. Expressing emotions: *is able to tell you how they are feeling and why (Qu 6)*		✓					✓
5. Understanding emotions: *is able to tell you two things that shows some insight into what makes them feel happy/sad or something that helps (Qu 7 & 8)*				✓			
SELF-ESTEEM							
6. Qualities and strengths: *is able to say three qualities/strengths about themselves (Qu 4, 9, 11 & 12)*				✓			
7. Self-esteem: *is able to talk positively about themselves and give at least three positive descriptors (All Questions)*			✓				
Completed by	SaLT						
Date	April 2022						

Name: WORKED EXAMPLE: Teenager

DoB: 16 years old

SELF-RATING SCALE							FORM 3
Please rate how easy or difficult you find the following							
Rating scale	**Very difficult** 1	2	3	4	5	**Very easy** 6	This is really important to me
1. Paying attention	1	2	3	(4)	5	6	
2. Making friends	1	(2)	3	4	5	6	✓
3. Playing with my friends	1	2	(3)	4	5	6	
4. Thinking of things that I like doing	1	2	3	(4)	5	6	
5. Thinking of things that I am good at	1	2	3	(4)	5	6	
6. Telling other people how I am feeling	(1)	2	3	4	5	6	✓
7. Knowing how someone else is feeling	1	2	(3)	4	5	6	
8. Coping with my feelings	1	(2)	3	4	5	6	
9. Feeling good about being me	1	2	(3)	4	5	6	✓
10. Looking at someone when I am talking to them	1	(2)	3	4	5	6	✓
11. Using body language	1	2	(3)	4	5	6	
12. Speaking clearly	1	2	3	4	(5)	6	
13. Listening to people	1	2	(3)	4	5	6	
14. Joining in conversations	(1)	2	3	4	5	6	✓
15. Taking turns in a conversation	1	(2)	3	4	5	6	
16. Answering questions	1	2	3	4	5	(6)	
17. Asking questions if I don't understand something	1	(2)	3	4	5	6	
18. Standing up for myself	1	(2)	3	4	5	6	

Thank you! Please now go back and choose the ones that are the most important to you.

Name: WORKED EXAMPLE: Teenager

DoB: 16 years old

SOCIAL SKILLS							FORM 4
Rating scale *Please rate the following in terms of appropriateness to the context:*	1 **Never**	2 **Rarely**	3 **Occasionally**	4 **Sometimes**	5 **Mostly**	6 **Always**	*Priority rating*
BODY LANGUAGE							
1. Eye contact		✓					✓
2. Facial expression		✓					✓
3. Use of hands/gesture		✓					
4. Distance/proximity				✓			
5. Use of touch				✓			
6. Use of fidgeting		✓					
7. Posture		✓					
8. Personal appearance					✓		
THE WAY WE TALK							
9. Volume			✓				
10. Rate				✓			
11. Clarity					✓		
12. Intonation			✓				
13. Fluency					✓		

Name: WORKED EXAMPLE: *Teenager*

DoB: *16 years old*

SOCIAL SKILLS 2.							**FORM 4**
Rating scale *Please rate the following in terms of appropriateness to the context:*	1 **Never**	2 **Rarely**	3 **Occasionally**	4 **Sometimes**	5 **Mostly**	6 **Always**	*Priority rating*
CONVERSATIONAL SKILLS							
14. Listening				✓			
15. Starting a conversation		✓					
16. Taking turns		✓					
17. Asking questions			✓				
18. Answering questions				✓			
19. Relevance			✓				
20. Repairing a breakdown			✓				
21. Ending a conversation			✓				

Name: WORKED EXAMPLE: *Teenager* DoB: 16 years old

SOCIAL SKILLS 3.							FORM 4
Rating scale *Please rate the following in terms of appropriateness to the context:*	1 **Never**	2 **Rarely**	3 **Occasionally**	4 **Sometimes**	5 **Mostly**	6 **Always**	Priority rating
ASSERTIVENESS							
22. Expressing feelings	✓						✓
23. Standing up for self or beliefs	✓						
24. Making suggestions or giving opinions			✓				
25. Refusing with reason/apology			✓				
26. Disagreeing with reason or compromise		✓					
27. Complaining with reason		✓					
28. Apologising shows remorse/ responsibility		✓					
29. Requesting explanations		✓					
Completed by	Mother/SaLT						
Date	April 2022						

TASS

Talkabout Assessment of Social Skills

Name: WorkedExample 16y

DoB: 11/05/2006

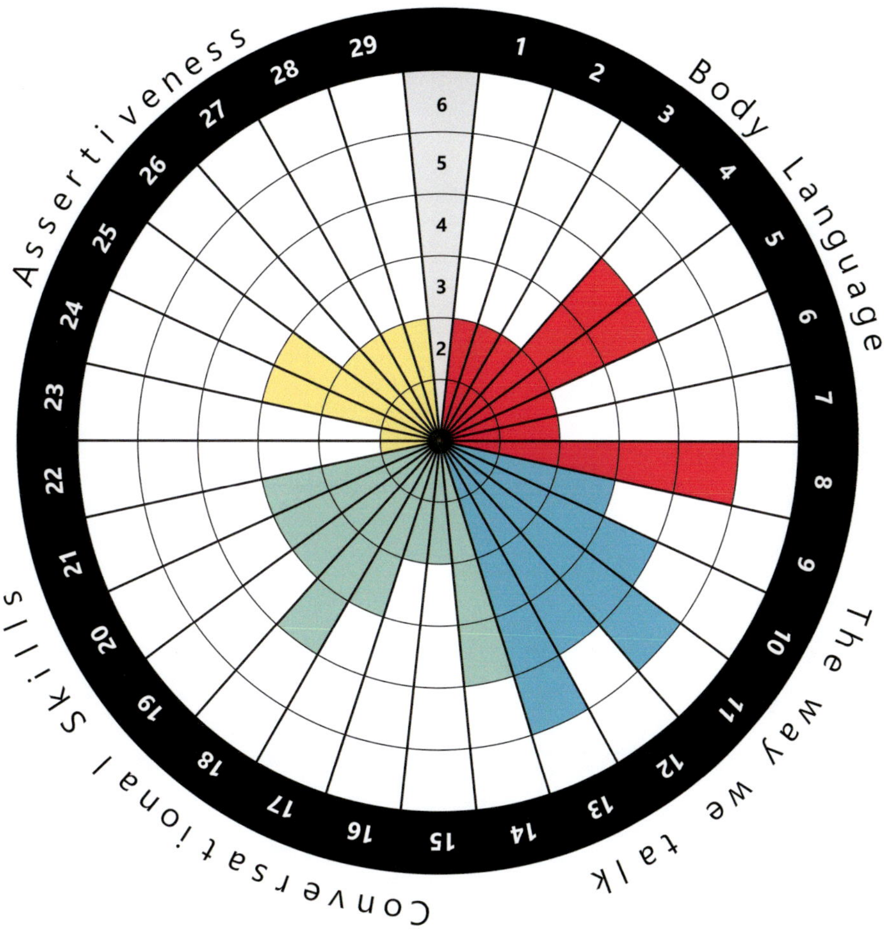

BODY LANGUAGE	THE WAY WE TALK	CONVERSATIONAL SKILLS	ASSERTIVENESS
1. Eye contact	9. Volume	14. Listening	22. Expressing feelings
2. Facial expression	10. Rate	15. Starting a conversation	23. Standing up for self
3. Gesture	11. Clarity	16. Taking turns	24. Making suggestions
4. Distance	12. Intonation	17. Asking questions	25. Refusing
5. Touch	13. Fluency	18. Answering questions	26. Disagreeing
6. Fidgeting		19. Relevance	27. Complaining
7. Posture		20. Repairing	28. Apologising
8. Personal appearance		21. Ending a conversation	29. Requesting explainations

Name: WORKED EXAMPLE: Child DoB: *9 years old*

INITIAL INFORMATION	**FORM 1**
A. PERSONAL INFORMATION	
Address	*Lives with parents*
Telephone number	
School/occupation	*Mainstream primary*
Contact at school	
Contact at home	
B. DESCRIPTION OF PERSON'S SOCIAL SKILLS	
Reason for referral	*Challenging behaviour*
Relevant diagnoses	*ASD traits and demand avoidance*
External factors which influence social skills (e.g., environmental, cultural, events)	*Masking at school*
Examples of situations the person finds difficult	*Transitioning between activities*
	Being asked to do something he doesn't want to
	Family dynamics

Name: WORKED EXAMPLE: Child

DoB: 9 years old

C. ASSOCIATED FACTORS							
Rating scale Please rate the following	1 Never	2 Rarely	3 Occasionally	4 Sometimes	5 Mostly	6 Always	Priority rating
1. Reaches expected academic goals				✓			
2. Demonstrates expected attention and listening skills			✓				
3. Manages internalised behaviours effectively *(e.g., withdrawal, anxiety)*		✓					
4. Manages externalised behaviours effectively *(e.g., aggression)*		✓					✓
5. Demonstrates cooperative behaviours *(e.g., sharing, following rules)*		✓					
6. Shows empathy		✓					
7. Able to regulate emotions		✓					✓
8. Able to problem solve		✓					
D. QUALITY OF LIFE							
1. Has healthy self-esteem			✓				✓
2. Has good mental health			✓				
3. Develops and maintains good relationships *(e.g., family, romantic)*					✓		
4. Develops and maintains friendships			✓				
5. Achieves occupational success *(e.g., school, higher education, employment – paid or voluntary)*					✓		

Name: WORKED EXAMPLE: *Child*

DoB: *9 years old*

E. ACTION PLAN	
Long-term goal Please describe what the person would like to achieve as a result of intervention.	*To be able to regulate emotions better and feel better about who he is.* *To help him see things from someone else's point of view* *To help him engage in activities/find things that interest him*
Any other comments	
Next steps	*Social skills group*
Person(s) completing form	*Mother*
Date	*March 2022*

Name: WORKED EXAMPLE: Child DoB: 9 years old

SELF-AWARENESS AND SELF-ESTEEM INTERVIEW	FORM 2	
1. Let's talk about some of the things you like doing. *Can you tell me three things you like or enjoy?* *Example prompts: favourite lesson; favourite game; hobbies or activities*	**Verbal Prompt?** √	**Visual Prompt?** √
1. Football 2. Maths 3. English	1. 2. 3.	1. 2. 3.
2. Is there anything you really don't like doing? *Can you think of three things you don't like or don't enjoy?* *Example prompts: lesson; game; hobbies or activities*		
1. Avocado 2. R.E. 3. Appointments	1. 2. 3.	1. 2. 3.
3. Let's talk about someone you know. Do you have a good friend? Or a teacher you like? *Can you tell me three things about them?* *Example prompts: what they look like; why you like them; what kind of person are they?*		
1. Tall 2. Curly hair 3. Glasses	1. 2. 3.	1. 2. 3.
4. What do you think that person would say about you? *Can you think of two things that they would say about you?* *Example prompts: what you look like; why they like you; what kind of person you are?*		
1. Self-conscious 2. Lazy	1. 2.	1. 2. ✓

Name: WORKED EXAMPLE: Child DoB: 9 years old

5. Let's talk about the way you look. *Can you tell me three things about the way you look?* *Example prompts: hair colour/length; height, eye colour; skin; clothing; you can use visual prompt 1*	**Verbal Prompt?** √	**Visual Prompt?** √
1. Blue eyes	1.	1. ✓
2. Brown hair	2.	2. ✓
3. Tall	3.	3. ✓
6. How are you feeling today? *Using the feelings board, can you tell me how you are feeling and why?* *Example prompts: are you happy; sad; worried or something else? use visual prompt 2 (feelings)*		
1. Bored, fed up, tired. Bored if I'm not on YouTube	1.	1. Feeling bored
7. Let's talk about your feelings more … *Can you think of something that makes you feel… happy? excited? sad? angry? worried?* *Example prompts: subjects at school; activities or hobbies*		
1. Happy or excited? YouTube	1.	1.
2. Sad, angry or worried? Bored if not on YouTube	2. ✓	2. ✓
8. What helps you when you are feeling sad, or angry or worried? *Can you think of anything that helps you?* *Example prompts: an activity or a person*		
1. YouTube	1. ✓	1. ✓
2.	2.	2.

Name: WORKED EXAMPLE: Child DoB: 9 years old

9. What are you good at? *Can you think of two things that you are good at?* *Example prompts: subjects at school; activities or hobbies*	**Verbal Prompt?** √	**Visual Prompt?** √
1. Maths 2. English 3. Running	1. ✓ 2. ✓	1. 2.
10. Is there anything that you find difficult? *Is there something that you find hard at school or home?* *Example prompts: subjects at school; activities or hobbies*		
1. Paying attention 2. Hard working	1. 2.	1. 2.
11. What kind of person do you think you are? *Can you think of three words to describe what you are like?* *Example prompts: chatty or quiet; hard-working or lazy; you can use visual prompt 3*		
1. Lazy	1. 2. 3.	1. ✓ 2. 3.
12. Tell me the best thing about being you. *Is there one thing you really like about being you?* *Example prompts: about themselves/their family; school; activities*		
1. Watching YouTube	1.	1.
13. If you could change one thing about being you, what would it be? *Example prompts: about themselves/their family; school; activities*		
1. Would like to be brave	1. ✓	1. ✓
14. Is there anything you would like to ask me? *I've asked you lots of questions, so is there anything you would like to ask me?*		
Nothing	1.	1.

Name: WORKED EXAMPLE: Child

DoB: 9 years old

SELF-AWARENESS AND SELF-ESTEEM SUMMARY — FORM 2

Rating scale	1 **No, never** *even with lots of support*	2 **Yes, but rarely** *and only with lots of support*	3 **Yes, occasionally** *or with some support*	4 **Yes, sometimes** *or in familiar situations only*	5 **Yes, mostly** *but not always*	6 **Yes, always**	*Priority rating*
SELF/OTHER AWARENESS							
1. Likes and dislikes: *is able to describe three things they like and three things they dislike (Qu 1 & 2)*				✓			
2. Other awareness: *is able to describe someone else using at least three descriptive words (Qu 3)*					✓		
3. Personal awareness: *is able to describe the way they look using at least three descriptive words (Qu 5)*					✓		
EMOTIONS							
4. Expressing emotions: *is able to tell you how they are feeling and why (Qu 6)*			✓				
5. Understanding emotions: *is able to tell you two things that shows some insight into what makes them feel happy/sad or something that helps (Qu 7 & 8)*		✓					
SELF-ESTEEM							
6. Qualities and strengths: *is able to say three qualities/strengths about themselves (Qu 4, 9, 11 & 12)*		✓					
7. Self-esteem: *is able to talk positively about themselves and give at least three positive descriptors (All Questions)*		✓					
Completed by	*SaLT*						
Date	*March 2022*						

Name: WORKED EXAMPLE: Child

DoB: 9 years old

SELF-RATING SCALE							FORM 3
Please rate how easy or difficult you find the following							
Rating scale	**Very difficult** 1	2	3	4	5	**→ Very easy** 6	This is really important to me
1. Paying attention	1	2	3	(4)	5	6	
2. Making friends	1	(2)	3	4	5	6	✓
3. Playing with my friends	1	2	(3)	4	5	6	
4. Thinking of things that I like doing	1	2	3	(4)	5	6	
5. Thinking of things that I am good at	1	2	3	(4)	5	6	
6. Telling other people how I am feeling	(1)	2	3	4	5	6	✓
7. Knowing how someone else is feeling	1	2	(3)	4	5	6	
8. Coping with my feelings	1	(2)	3	4	5	6	
9. Feeling good about being me	1	2	(3)	4	5	6	✓
10. Looking at someone when I am talking to them	1	(2)	3	4	5	6	✓
11. Using body language	1	2	(3)	4	5	6	
12. Speaking clearly	1	2	3	4	(5)	6	
13. Listening to people	1	2	(3)	4	5	6	
14. Joining in conversations	(1)	2	3	4	5	6	✓
15. Taking turns in a conversation	1	(2)	3	4	5	6	
16. Answering questions	1	2	3	4	5	(6)	
17. Asking questions if I don't understand something	1	(2)	3	4	5	6	
18. Standing up for myself	1	(2)	3	4	5	6	

Thank you! Please now go back and choose the ones that are the most important to you.

Name: WORKED EXAMPLE: Child

DoB: 9 years old

SOCIAL SKILLS							FORM 4
Rating scale *Please rate the following in terms of appropriateness to the context:*	1 **Never**	2 **Rarely**	3 **Occasionally**	4 **Sometimes**	5 **Mostly**	6 **Always**	Priority rating
BODY LANGUAGE							
1. Eye contact					✓		✓
2. Facial expression					✓		✓
3. Use of hands/gesture					✓		
4. Distance/proximity			✓				
5. Use of touch			✓				
6. Use of fidgeting			✓				
7. Posture				✓			
8. Personal appearance				✓			
THE WAY WE TALK							
9. Volume					✓		
10. Rate				✓			
11. Clarity					✓		
12. Intonation					✓		
13. Fluency					✓		

Name: WORKED EXAMPLE: Child

DoB: 9 years old

SOCIAL SKILLS 2.							FORM 4
Rating scale *Please rate the following in terms of appropriateness to the context:*	1 **Never**	2 **Rarely**	3 **Occasionally**	4 **Sometimes**	5 **Mostly**	6 **Always**	Priority rating
CONVERSATIONAL SKILLS							
14. Listening				✓			
15. Starting a conversation			✓				
16. Taking turns			✓				✓
17. Asking questions		✓					
18. Answering questions				✓			
19. Relevance			✓				
20. Repairing a breakdown		✓					
21. Ending a conversation			✓				

Name: WORKED EXAMPLE: Child

DoB: 9 years old

SOCIAL SKILLS 3.							FORM 4
Rating scale *Please rate the following in terms of appropriateness to the context:*	1 **Never**	2 **Rarely**	3 **Occasionally**	4 **Sometimes**	5 **Mostly**	6 **Always**	Priority rating
ASSERTIVENESS							
22. Expressing feelings		✓					✓
23. Standing up for self or beliefs		✓					
24. Making suggestions or giving opinions		✓					
25. Refusing with reason/apology		✓					✓
26. Disagreeing with reason or compromise		✓					✓
27. Complaining with reason		✓					✓
28. Apologising shows remorse/ responsibility		✓					
29. Requesting explanations		✓					
Completed by	Mother/SaLT						
Date	March 2022						

TASS

Talkabout Assessment of Social Skills

Name: WorkedExample 9y

DoB: 29/04/2013

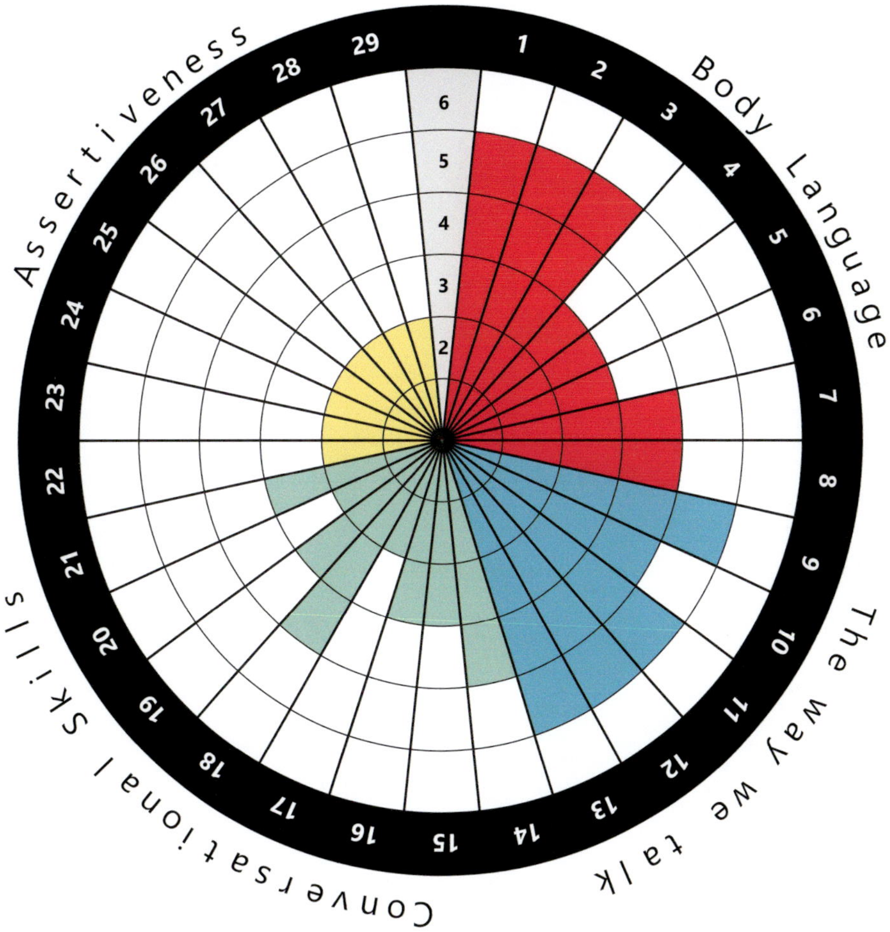

BODY LANGUAGE	THE WAY WE TALK	CONVERSATIONAL SKILLS	ASSERTIVENESS
1. Eye contact	9. Volume	14. Listening	22. Expressing feelings
2. Facial expression	10. Rate	15. Starting a conversation	23. Standing up for self
3. Gesture	11. Clarity	16. Taking turns	24. Making suggestions
4. Distance	12. Intonation	17. Asking questions	25. Refusing
5. Touch	13. Fluency	18. Answering questions	26. Disagreeing
6. Fidgeting		19. Relevance	27. Complaining
7. Posture		20. Repairing	28. Apologising
8. Personal appearance		21. Ending a conversation	29. Requesting explainations

Name: .... DoB: ....

INITIAL INFORMATION	FORM 1
A. PERSONAL INFORMATION	
Address	
Telephone number	
School/occupation	
Contact at school	
Contact at home	
B. DESCRIPTION OF PERSON'S SOCIAL SKILLS	
Reason for referral	
Relevant diagnoses	
External factors which influence social skills *(e.g., environmental, cultural, events)*	
Examples of situations the person finds difficult	1.
	2.
	3.

Name: .... DoB: ....

C. ASSOCIATED FACTORS							
Rating scale Please rate the following	1 Never	2 Rarely	3 Occasionally	4 Sometimes	5 Mostly	6 Always	Priority rating
1. Reaches expected academic goals							
2. Demonstrates expected attention and listening skills							
3. Manages internalised behaviours effectively *(e.g., anxiety)*							
4. Manages externalised behaviours effectively *(e.g., aggression)*							
5. Demonstrates cooperative behaviours *(e.g., sharing, following rules)*							
6. Shows empathy							
7. Able to regulate emotions							
8. Able to problem solve							
D. QUALITY OF LIFE							
1. Has healthy self-esteem							
2. Has good mental health							
3. Develops and maintains close relationships *(e.g., family, romantic)*							
4. Develops and maintains friendships							
5. Achieves occupational success *(e.g., school, higher ed., paid/unpaid employment)*							

Name: ....

DoB: ....

E. ACTION PLAN	
Long-term goal *Please describe what the person would like to achieve as a result of intervention.*	
Any other comments	
Next steps	
Person(s) completing form	
Date	

Name: .... DoB: ....

SELF-AWARENESS AND SELF-ESTEEM INTERVIEW		**FORM 2**
1. Let's talk about some of the things you like doing. *Can you tell me three things you like or enjoy?* *Example prompts: favourite lesson; favourite game; hobbies or activities*	***Verbal Prompt?*** √	***Visual Prompt?*** √
1.	1.	1.
2.	2.	2.
3.	3.	3.
2. Is there anything you really don't like doing? *Can you think of three things you don't like or don't enjoy?* *Example prompts: lesson; game; hobbies or activities*		
1.	1.	1.
2.	2.	2.
3.	3.	3.
3. Let's talk about someone you know. Do you have a good friend? Or a teacher you like? *Can you tell me three things about them?* *Example prompts: what they look like; why you like them; what kind of person are they?*		
1.	1.	1.
2.	2.	2.
3.	3.	3.
4. What do you think that person would say about you? *Can you think of two things that they would say about you?* *Example prompts: what you look like; why they like you; what kind of person you are?*		
1.	1.	1.
2.	2.	2.

Name: ....   DoB: ....

5. Let's talk about the way you look. *Can you tell me three things about the way you look?* *Example prompts: hair colour/length; height, eye colour; skin; clothing; you can use visual prompt 1*	**Verbal Prompt?** √	**Visual Prompt?** √
1. 2. 3.	1. 2. 3.	1. 2. 3.
6. How are you feeling today? *Using the feelings board, can you tell me how you are feeling and why?* *Example prompts: are you happy; sad; worried or something else? use visual prompt 2 (feelings)*		
1.	1.	1. Feelings board
7. Let's talk about your feelings more … *Can you think of something that makes you feel … happy? excited? sad? angry? worried?* *Example prompts: subjects at school; activities or hobbies*		
1. Happy or excited? 2. Sad, angry or worried?	1. 2.	1. 2.
8. What helps you when you are feeling sad, or angry or worried? *Can you think of anything that helps you?* *Example prompts: an activity or a person*		
1. 2.	1. 2.	1. 2.

Name: .... DoB: ....

9. What are you good at? *Can you think of two things that you are good at?* *Example prompts: subjects at school; activities or hobbies*	**Verbal Prompt?** √	**Visual Prompt?** √
1. 2.	1. 2.	1. 2.

10. Is there anything that you find difficult? *Is there something that you find hard at school or home?* *Example prompts: subjects at school; activities or hobbies*		
1. 2.	1. 2.	1. 2.

11. What kind of person do you think you are? *Can you think of three words to describe what you are like?* *Example prompts: chatty or quiet; hard-working or lazy; you can use visual prompt 3*		
1. 2. 3.	1. 2. 3.	1. 2. 3.

12. Tell me the best thing about being you. *Is there one thing you really like about being you?* *Example prompts: about themselves/their family; school; activities*		
1.	1.	1.

13. If you could change one thing about being you, what would it be? *Example prompts: about themselves/their family; school; activities*		
1.	1.	1.

14. Is there anything you would like to ask me? *I've asked you lots of questions, so is there anything you would like to ask me?*		
1.	1.	1.

Name: .... DoB: ....

SELF-AWARENESS AND SELF-ESTEEM SUMMARY — FORM 2

Rating scale	1 **No, never** even with lots of support	2 **Yes, but *rarely*** *and* only with lots of support	3 **Yes, occasionally** or with some support	4 **Yes, sometimes** or in familiar situations only	5 **Yes, mostly** but not always	6 **Yes, *always***	Priority rating
SELF/OTHER AWARENESS							
1. Likes and dislikes: is able to describe three things they like and three things they dislike (Qu 1 & 2)							
2. Other awareness: is able to describe someone else using at least three descriptive words (Qu 3)							
3. Personal awareness: is able to describe the way they look using at least three descriptive words (Qu 5)							
EMOTIONS							
4. Expressing emotions: is able to tell you how they are feeling and why (Qu 6)							
5. Understanding emotions: is able to tell you two things that shows some insight into what makes them feel happy/sad or something that helps (Qu 7 & 8)							
SELF-ESTEEM							
6. Qualities and strengths: is able to say three qualities/strengths about themselves (Qu 4, 9, 11 & 12)							
7. Self-esteem: is able to talk positively about themselves and give at least three positive descriptors (All Questions)							
Completed by							
Date							

Name: .... DoB: ....

SELF-RATING SCALE							FORM 3
Please rate how easy or difficult you find the following							
Rating scale	**Very difficult → Very easy** 1	2	3	4	5	6	This is really important to me
1. Paying attention	1	2	3	4	5	6	
2. Making friends	1	2	3	4	5	6	
3. Playing with my friends	1	2	3	4	5	6	
4. Thinking of things that I like doing	1	2	3	4	5	6	
5. Thinking of things that I am good at	1	2	3	4	5	6	
6. Telling other people how I am feeling	1	2	3	4	5	6	
7. Knowing how someone else is feeling	1	2	3	4	5	6	
8. Coping with my feelings	1	2	3	4	5	6	
9. Feeling good about being me	1	2	3	4	5	6	
10. Looking at someone when I am talking to them	1	2	3	4	5	6	
11. Using body language	1	2	3	4	5	6	
12. Speaking clearly	1	2	3	4	5	6	
13. Listening to people	1	2	3	4	5	6	
14. Joining in conversations	1	2	3	4	5	6	
15. Taking turns in a conversation	1	2	3	4	5	6	
16. Answering questions	1	2	3	4	5	6	
17. Asking questions if I don't understand something	1	2	3	4	5	6	
18. Standing up for myself	1	2	3	4	5	6	

Thank you! Please now go back and choose the ones that are the most important to you.

Name: .... DoB: ....

SOCIAL SKILLS							FORM 4
Rating scale *Please rate the following in terms of appropriateness to the context:*	1 **Never**	2 **Rarely**	3 **Occasionally**	4 **Sometimes**	5 **Mostly**	6 **Always**	Priority rating
BODY LANGUAGE							
1. Eye contact							
2. Facial expression							
3. Use of hands/gesture							
4. Distance/proximity							
5. Use of touch							
6. Use of fidgeting							
7. Posture							
8. Personal appearance							
THE WAY WE TALK							
9. Volume							
10. Rate							
11. Clarity							
12. Intonation							
13. Fluency							

Name: ....

DoB: ....

SOCIAL SKILLS 2.							FORM 4
Rating scale *Please rate the following in terms of appropriateness to the context:*	1 **Never**	2 **Rarely**	3 **Occasionally**	4 **Sometimes**	5 **Mostly**	6 **Always**	Priority rating
CONVERSATIONAL SKILLS							
14. Listening							
15. Starting a conversation							
16. Taking turns							
17. Asking questions							
18. Answering questions							
19. Relevance							
20. Repairing a breakdown							
21. Ending a conversation							

Name: .... DoB: ....

SOCIAL SKILLS 3.							FORM 4
Rating scale *Please rate the following in terms of appropriateness to the context:*	1 **Never**	2 **Rarely**	3 **Occasionally**	4 **Sometimes**	5 **Mostly**	6 **Always**	Priority rating
ASSERTIVENESS							
22. Expressing feelings							
23. Standing up for self or beliefs							
24. Making suggestions or giving opinions							
25. Refusing with reason/apology							
26. Disagreeing with reason or compromise							
27. Complaining with reason							
28. Apologising shows remorse/ responsibility							
29. Requesting explanations							
Completed by							
Date							

What do you look like? (1)

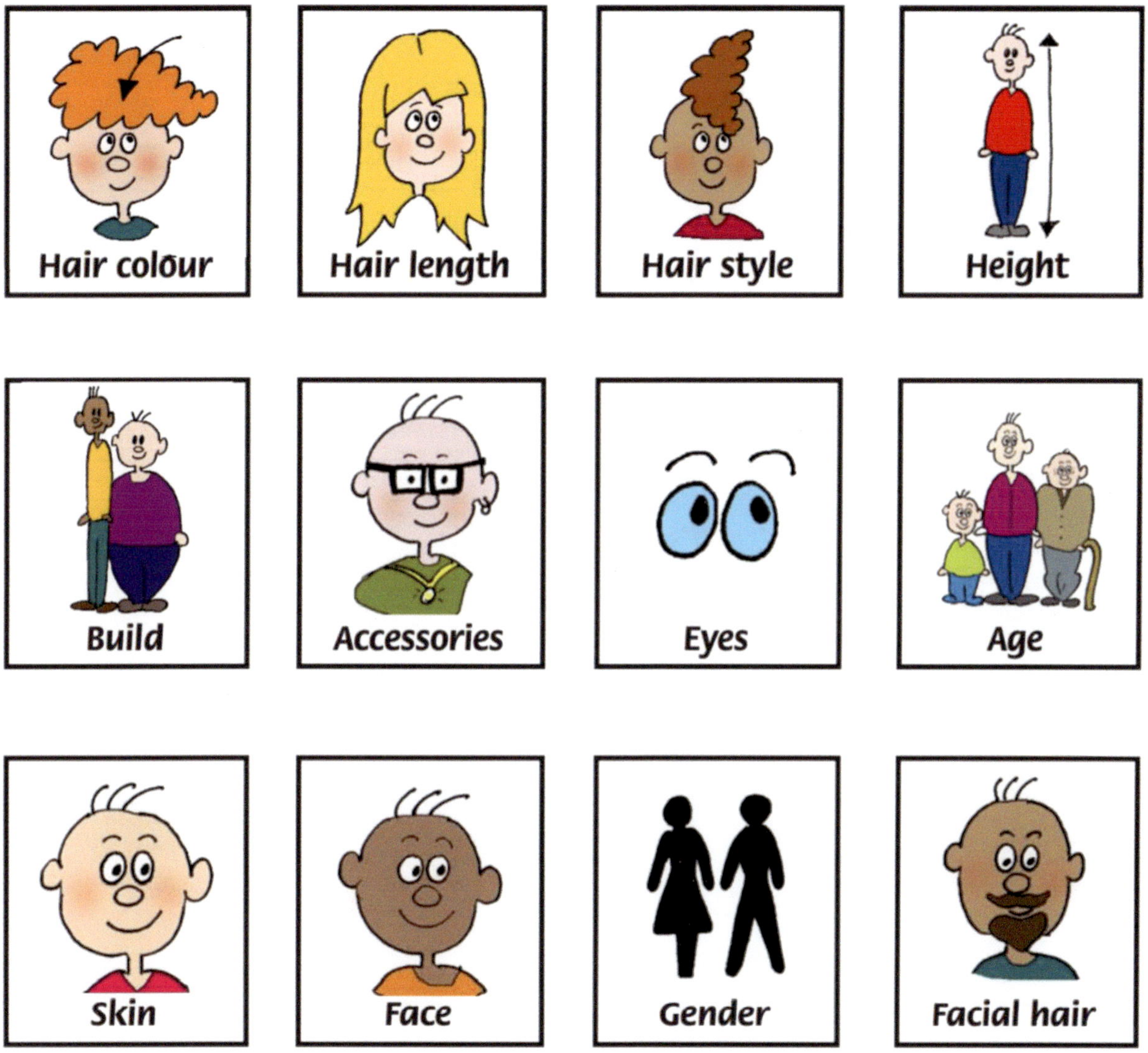

Prompt 1 Question 5

What do you look like? (2)

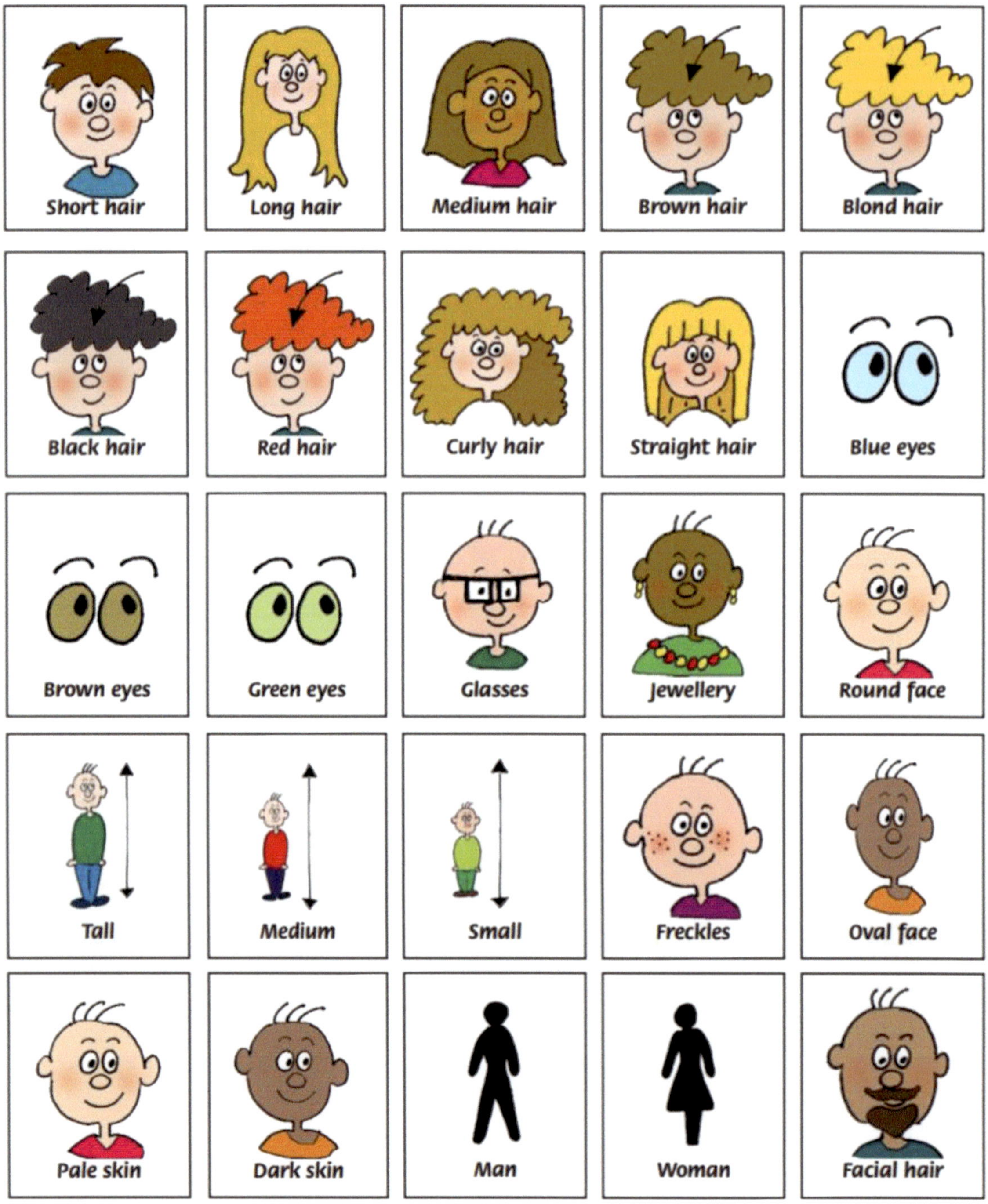

Prompt 1 Question 5

How are you feeling? (1)

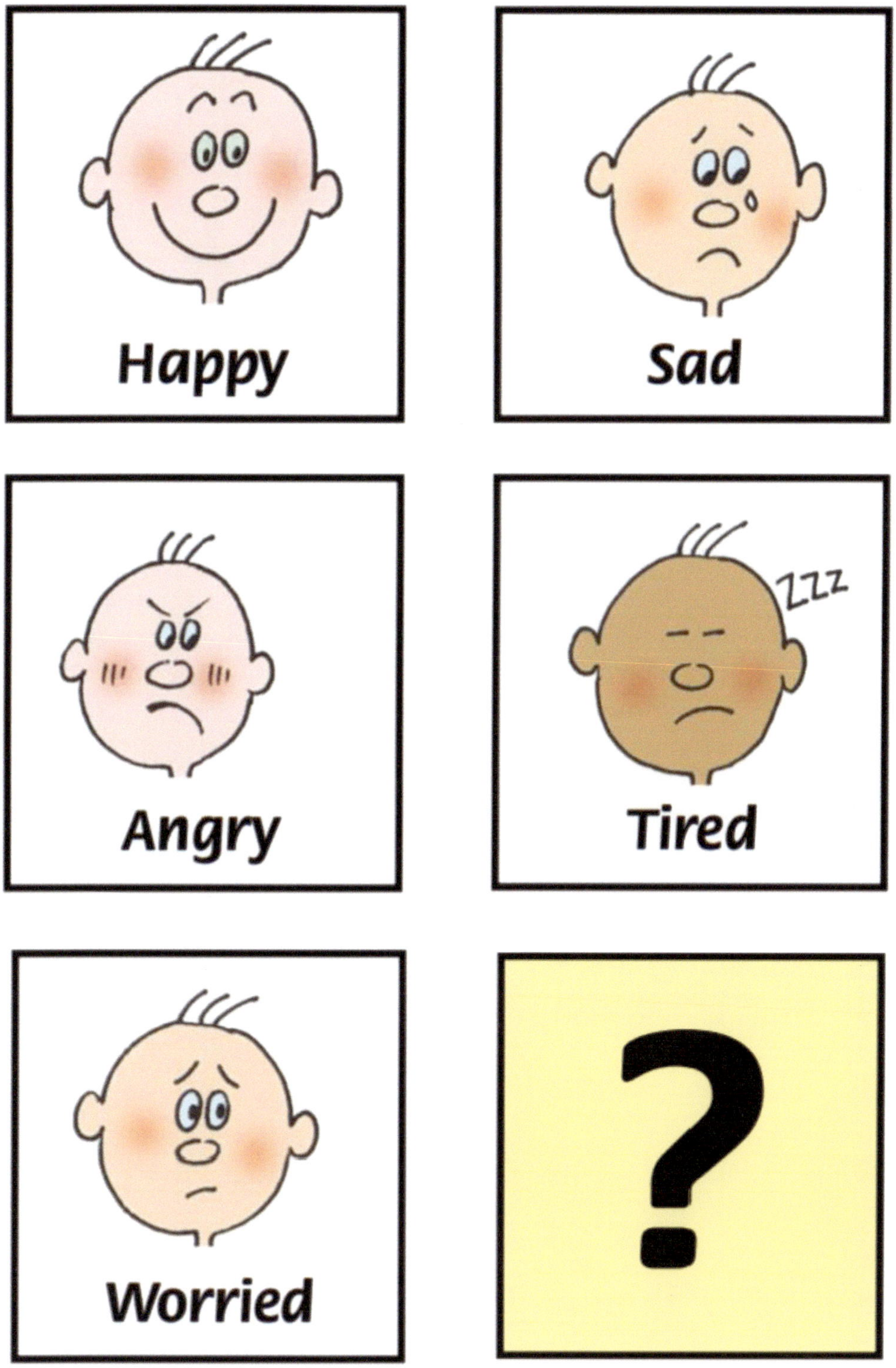

Prompt 2 Question 6

How are you feeling? (2)

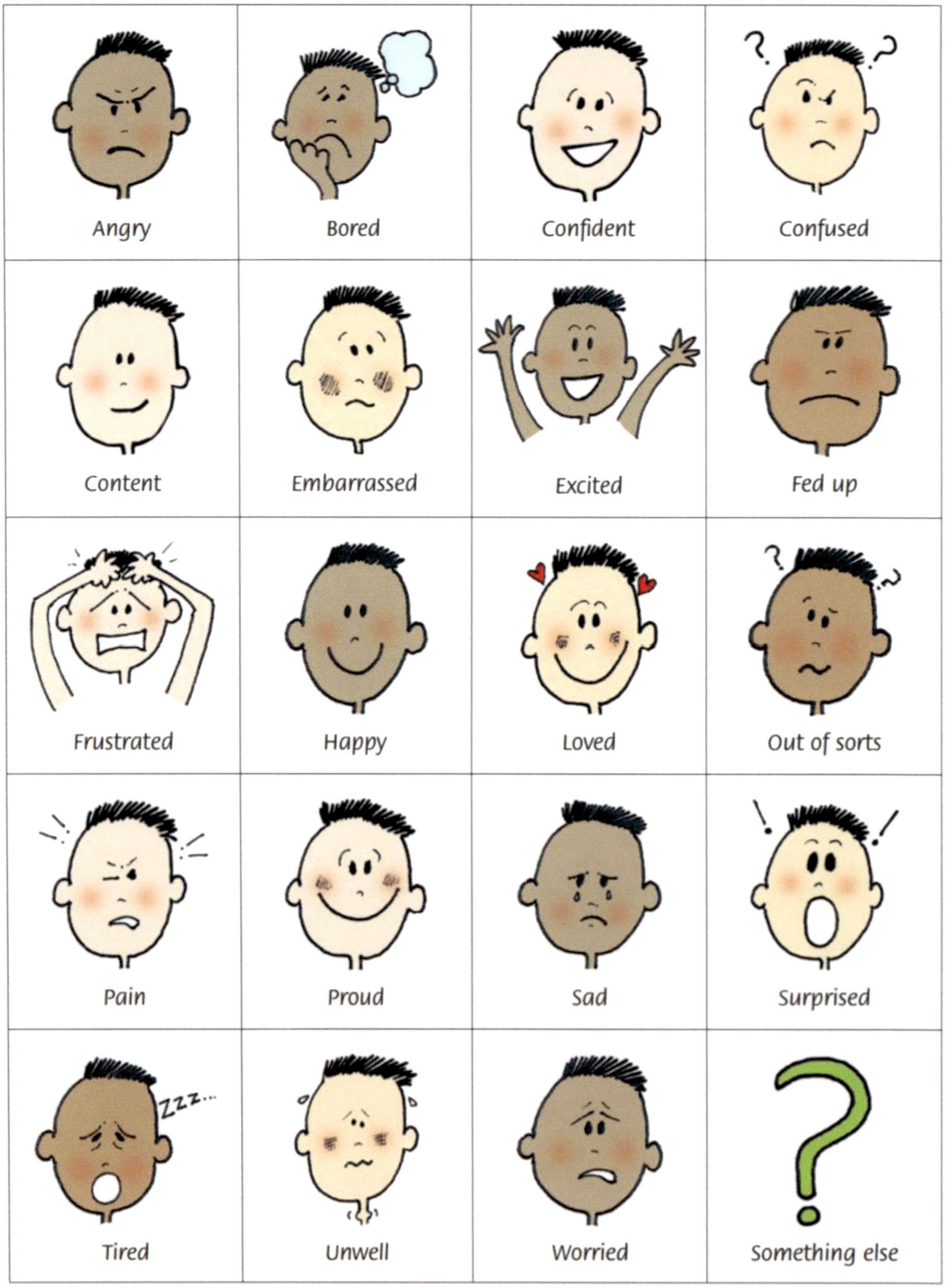

Prompt 2 Question 6

What are you like?

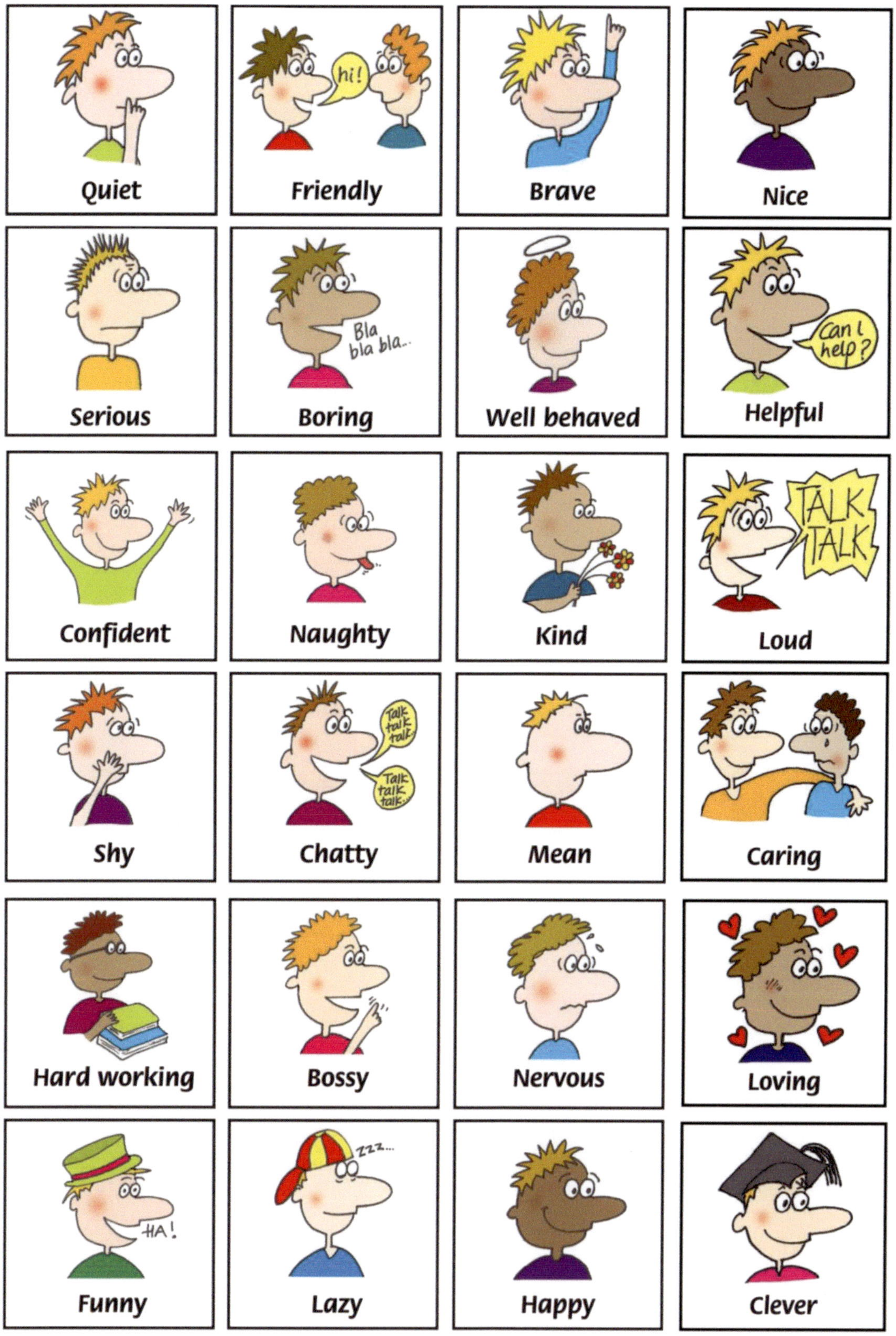

Prompt 3 Question 11